Praise fo.
The Power of Positive Aging

"One of the best books I have read on wellness and aging for a long time. On a scale of 1 to 10, I give it a big 10."
—**Larry W. Hayes,** *Active After 50*

"David Lereah takes us on a personal journey for the ages; his battle against stage three cancer. Along the way he discovers the power of positive aging and presents his findings in this book. It is an inspiring story of how a positive mindset can overcome the physical and mental challenges of aging and disease. A must-read for anyone over 50 years old."
—**Chip Conley,** founder of Modern Elder Academy, *New York Times* best selling author, and Next Avenue's 2019 Top Ten Influencer in Aging

"*The Power of Positive Aging* is an essential resource for anyone facing the prospect of older age. David Lereah adeptly shows how aging does not have to be the negative experience we've been taught it is."
—**Lawrence R. Samuel,** author of *Aging in America* and *Boomers 3.0* and Next Avenue's 2017 Top Ten Influencer in Aging

"If you're a baby boomer, this indispensable guide needs to be in your personal library. Filled with spiritual insights, practical tools, and helpful resources, you will return to it time and again as you navigate the uncharted territory of your own unique journey into older age. Kudos to David Lereah for infusing each page with both extensive research and the wisdom of one who knows whereof he speaks."
—**Mary Eileen Williams,** host of the *Feisty Side of Fifty* podcast

"A supportive and practical guide for positive aging. This brilliant and engaging book embodies wisdom, personal insights, as well as the tools we all need for facing life's greatest challenge. A true inspiration."
—**Susan Landeis,** author of *Optimal Caregiving*

"*The Power of Positive Aging* takes us on a different path to aging that is profoundly productive for ourselves and others. Aging is the greatest education about life a person can have, and David Lereah has laid out all the study tools needed to graduate with high honors. David shows us a path that changes aging from a challenge to an experience. It is a masterful collection of tools—physical, mental and spiritual—that enable us to craft our own path through the aging process."
—**Lee Mowatt,** vlogger, senior fitness motivator, and host of *The Aging Academy* podcast

"*The Power of Positive Aging* is not just another feel-good book about growing older. Driven by David Lereah's personal journey with cancer and its aftermath, this book is a guide for creating a positive framework for leading life as we age. He examines inner spirit, social networks, and emotional intelligence in a thoughtful way. Particularly insightful is his chapter "Reclaim Your Life" and his advice on creating a lifestyle plan for positive aging. An easy read and very insightful, this is a must-read as you embrace this stage of life and positive message that we need now more than ever due to the coronavirus pandemic."
—**Lori Bitter,** The Business of Aging, author of *The Grandparent Economy*, and Next Avenue's 2017 Top Influencer in Aging

"David Lereah's book *The Power of Positive Aging* is an important contribution to help meet the challenges of aging. You will learn the mental and spiritual strategies that he used to personally overcome his big challenge to emerge healthier and happier as he ages positively. His concept that the challenges that come with aging are just inconveniences, is one we all should embrace."
—**Rico Caveglia**, author of *Ageless Living* and host of the *Fearless Aging* podcast

"David Lereah's book *The Power of Positive Aging* provides a no-nonsense, fact-based approach to tackling the challenges of aging with grace and dignity. A cancer survivor himself, his reflections enhance the reader's understanding of how growing old comes with 'inconveniences.' This informative how-to guide provides instructions and solutions for his vision of aging positively while at the same time fostering an age-friendly society that will benefit anyone who reads it."
—**Angela G. Gentile**, MSW, RSW

"Full of hard-won wisdom. David Lereah has written a personal, practical and comprehensive book on how to accept the challenges of aging, while enjoying the richness of the present moment. The book is well researched and full of great examples of how to live your best life until the very last breath. I love the concept of 'the inconvenience of aging'—it puts the process into real perspective."
—**Nicole Christina**, LCSW, psychotherapist, and host of the *Zestful Aging* podcast

The Power of Positive Aging

Successfully Coping with the Inconveniences of Aging

David Alan Lereah, PhD

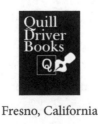

Fresno, California

Published by Quill Driver Books
An imprint of Linden Publishing
2006 South Mary Street, Fresno, California 93721
(559) 233-6633 / (800) 345-4447
QuillDriverBooks.com

Quill Driver Books and Colophon are trademarks of
Linden Publishing, Inc.

cover design by Tanja Prokop, www.bookcoverworld.com
interior design by Andrea Reider

ISBN 978-1-61035-360-1

135798642

Printed in the United States of America
on acid-free paper.

Library of Congress Cataloging-in-Publication Data

Names: Lereah, David A., author.
Title: The power of positive aging : successfully coping with the
   inconveniences of aging / David Lereah, PhD.
Identifiers: LCCN 2020021692 (print) | LCCN 2020021693 (ebook) |
ISBN
   9781610353601 (paperback) | ISBN 9781610353724 (kindle edition) |
ISBN
   9781610353724 (epub)
Subjects: LCSH: Aging--Social aspects--United States. | Self-realization in
   old age--United States. | Older people--Care--United States. | Quality
   of life--United States. | Mindfulness (Psychology)--United States.
Classification: LCC HQ1064.U5 .L467 2020 (print) | LCC HQ1064.U5
(ebook)
   | DDC 305.260973--dc23
LC record available at https://lccn.loc.gov/2020021692
LC ebook record available at https://lccn.loc.gov/2020021693

Contents

"I do not fear death. I had been dead for billions and billions of years before I was born and had not suffered the slightest inconvenience from it."

—MARK TWAIN

Introduction
Growing Old Is a
New Phenomenon

It may come as a surprise to many, but growing old is a relatively new phenomenon. We are living almost thirty years longer than the longevity numbers of just 100 years ago. People who lived only to age 49 or 50 died before their bodies experienced many of the marks of aging most of us face today, like hearing impairment, loss of mobility, and dementia.

For 99.9 percent of the time humans have inhabited the Earth, average life expectancy topped out at thirty to forty years. In 1900, the average life span in the United States was forty-seven years. Just over a century later, the average life span has skyrocketed to almost seventy-nine years. For older age groups, life spans are even longer. If you are 65, your life expectancy is eighty-four years.

A silver tsunami is sweeping America. More than 10,000 people per day in the United States are turning 65. The senior population—those 65 and older—is projected to reach 88.5 million by 2050. That is more than double the population of 39.6 million seniors in 2010. By 2050, at least 400,000 seniors will be 100 or older.[1]

Aging Occurs Throughout Our Lifetimes

Aging doesn't just happen when we reach 65; it begins in our 20s. According to Robert Kail and John Cavanaugh, sensory abilities peak in your early 20s. Hearing begins to decline by your late 20s, while vision typically begins to deteriorate in middle age. The muscle strength in men and women peaks between 20 and 30, and resting metabolism, which accounts for a major part of daily energy consumption, peaks in early adulthood. According to Valerie Gladwell, your endurance peaks at age 22, while memory peaks at 28.[2]

Suffice it to say that we are physically and mentally deteriorating for the majority of our lifetimes. But for most of us, aging doesn't begin to have a significant impact on the quality of our lives until after we pass 50.

Learning How to Age

Most of us begin life believing we are immortal and assuming that nothing bad will happen to us. As we grow old and encounter the physical and mental hallmarks of aging, the reality of our mortality and the concept of finality creeps into our thoughts. Time marches on; there is no slowing life.

Although all of us are aging, few of us are prepared to deal with its realities. No one teaches us how to deal with wrinkles, loss of mobility, or fading eyesight, and certainly no one prepares us to deal with life-threatening diseases. Moreover, trying to age gracefully and with dignity, feels like swimming against the tide of today's forever-young society, where the young are perceived as beautiful and energetic while the old are seen as stale and useless.

In this society, wrinkles are ugly, and wheelchairs represent helplessness. No wonder many seniors are ashamed or embarrassed to display marks of aging, and no wonder more than 6.5 million seniors in America are diagnosed with some form of depression.[3] Like golf-ball-sized hail coming at us with a reckless abandon, every mark of aging can chip away at our self-worth.

But we don't have to measure our self-worth by our youthful skin tone or our ability to run marathons. Aging—and its accompanying physical and mental challenges—may be inevitable, but our later years do not have to be miserable. How we effectively cope with serious physical and mental decline is the raison d'être for this book and is the subject this book's comprehensive program addresses. As a cancer survivor, I have discovered the extraordinary power of practicing positive aging, and I want to share this recipe for experiencing a more joyful life in your senior years.

It is important to emphasize that practicing positive aging can begin at any age and is especially beneficial for people over 50 years old when serious age-related decline becomes a reality.

CHAPTER ONE

Why Positive Aging?

At 63 years old, I looked in the mirror and saw a thin and drawn face with a hopeless and almost vacant demeanor. I saw loose skin bundling below my chin. My self-worth was eroding by the day.

I was petrified about my life. I had survived stage 3 esophageal cancer and was now one of the walking wounded. The aftermath left me thirty pounds underweight, precariously living off a feeding tube, and incessantly coughing and gagging throughout the day. Further, my mind often felt foggy and was no longer the spry tool it once was. I was aging rapidly and didn't know how to cope with my sudden physical and mental decline.

I realized that everything I had learned and done with my life was no longer a "fit" in my altered state of existence. Of course, my doctor's solution was for me to see a psychiatrist. He believed I was deeply depressed about my post-surgery life, and thought I needed psychiatric therapy sessions to help me better cope with my new normal.

I ignored his diagnosis and prescription and took another route. I embarked on a journey of discovery and I found the power of positive aging. I came to understand that positive aging is a way of living life—a combination of developing certain mindset changes and physical and spiritual improvements—that I believe is a genuine solution to successful aging. It literally saved my life by helping me cope under the most trying conditions.

I'm convinced that the practice of positive aging is destined to enhance quality of life for everyone facing the marks of aging—whether it's a serious life-threatening disease like cancer; or a disease that lowers quality of life like arthritis and diabetes; or a mark of physical decline like mobility and hearing loss; or a mark of mental decline like dementia.

But before we go knee deep into the practice of positive aging, let's define what it means to achieve "successful aging" and how positive aging gets us there.

Successful Aging

Everyone wants to age successfully, but what is meant by "successful"? This question has been the subject of research for decades. However, the discussion over successful aging takes on greater importance today because the large baby boomer population is becoming senior citizens at a rapid pace and enjoying—along with everybody else—a significant improvement in life expectancy numbers.

Fortunately, doctors Elizabeth Phelan and Eric Larson conducted a review of over four decades of successful aging literature in order to present a consensus definition.[4] Later, working with two colleagues, they expanded on the previous study.[5] From the literature identified, they presented nine major elements of successful aging:

1. Life satisfaction
2. Longevity
3. Freedom from disability
4. Mastery/growth
5. Active engagement with life
6. High/independent functioning
7. Positive adaptation
8. Psychological health
9. The importance of interpersonal relationships

In summary, successful aging refers to a multidimensional involvement with life that is inclusive of physical, functional, psychological, and social health.

Based on my own experience, I would add a tenth element to the definition of successful aging:

10. Spiritual health

Positive Aging

While the literature is filled with different versions and meanings of positive aging, and while there is no set definition of positive aging across cultures and nations, there is universal agreement that growing older has a psychological impact on us. In general, positive aging covers our ability to maintain a positive attitude, stay in the present moment, feel confident about ourselves, keep fit and healthy, and engage fully in life.

That's why I believe that positive aging embodies all ten of the elements of successful aging. When embraced with enthusiasm, positive aging *becomes* successful aging, and allows us to write a fulfilling final chapter to our lives.

As we age, the practice of positive aging helps us better control our ability to cope with physical and mental decline. It also provides us with the wherewithal to fight off the stereotypes of ageism that could erode our self-worth.

Simply stated, positive aging is adopting a positive mindset of aging as a natural way of life. Rather than viewing aging in a negative light as something to be endured, aging is viewed as a positive journey of transition. Positive aging encompasses the elements of psychological, spiritual, physical, and social support. And beyond practicing positivity and holding a positive mindset, it also includes all the other beneficial things someone does because they are in a positive frame of mind, such as exercise, healthy diet, social interaction, and so on.

So, as you will see throughout this book, I set out on a journey to cope with the horrors of my cancer battle, and on the way I discovered useful notions and techniques that introduced me to the practice of positive aging. You will see boxes labeled "My Journey" scattered in subsequent chapters to demonstrate how I applied positive aging practices to my encounter with cancer.

I've come to believe that positive aging is a belief system that helps individuals better cope with the inconveniences one experiences throughout the aging process. The system's emphasis on an individual's psychological and spiritual health, as well as on developing and maintaining meaningful interpersonal relationships, creates a powerful defense system against the inevitable slings and arrows that life throws at us as we age.

The positive aging movement—led by educators such as Jan Hively, Encore.org; Meg Newhouse, Life Planning Network; and Dorian Mintzer, Revolutionize Retirement.org—is growing rapidly, and there is no shortage of research on it. Literally hundreds of articles and studies have been written on the subject (see Appendix C: Information Sources for Practicing Positive Aging). For a thorough review of the literature on positive aging, including theories of positive aging and the principles and philosophies behind it, see Kori Miller's article at Positive Psychology.com.[6]

Information about positive aging can also be found at places such as the Center for Positive Aging, in Atlanta, Georgia: CenterforPositiveAging.org. The Center exists to assist elders connect to the resources they need, and to educate consumers about the types of services available to assist in successful, positive aging. The Mather Institute is another organization focused on positive aging, sharing research, trends, and best practices (visit www.matherinstitute.com).

Another important goal of the positive aging movement is to counter and oppose the age-biased beliefs of ageism. One example is the article "Old Age Appreciated: The Positive Aging Movement," by Ruth Mutzner, PhD (PioneerNetwork.net, September 19, 2017). Of course, there are numerous organizations speaking out against ageism, including the Administration of Aging, AARP, American Society on Aging, Gerontology Society of America, and the National Institute on Aging.

The Benefits of Positive Aging

There are obviously a number of major benefits of practicing positive aging, notably enhanced physical, mental, emotional, and spiritual health. More specifically, individuals practicing positive aging will also likely become:

➢ More proactive about health
➢ More resilient to illness, enjoying improved immunity
➢ Less stressed-out, reducing their likelihood of developing chronic diseases or disorders
➢ More in touch with their spirit
➢ Practitioners of a healthier lifestyle
➢ More energetic

And perhaps most important of all, they will experience greater happiness and joy.

All these benefits clearly suggest that the greatest gain of practicing positive aging is to improve your overall quality of life as you age. A positive aging mindset will help you better cope with the onslaught of the marks of aging that you will confront throughout your senior years. A positive aging journey will contribute enormously to your happiness, so you can enjoy a richer, more satisfying life in your senior years.

The Science of Positive Aging

Positive aging is strongly supported by the science of aging. Not only will positive aging help you better cope with the marks of aging and the transition to getting older, but from a biological perspective, positive aging may indeed enhance life expectancy and lessen the likelihood of disease and other ailments. Positive aging means that not only will you cope better with the marks of aging and improve the quality of your life, but you will likely live a longer, healthier life.

A 2019 study asserts that positive thinking (a key element of positive aging) can result in an 11 to 15 percent longer life span and a stronger likelihood of living to age 85 or older. This effect remained after other factors such as age, gender, income, depression, and health status were controlled.[7]

The study indicates that optimistic individuals tend to have a reduced risk of depression, heart disease, and other chronic diseases. But optimism also might be linked to exceptional longevity. Optimistic people might be more motivated to try to maintain good health habits and practices, such as maintaining a decent diet, engaging in regular exercise, and not smoking. And they are better at regulating stress. All these factors are positively correlated with longevity.

This revelation claims that stress-free positive aging attitudes will lengthen life and make it more joyful in your senior years. But there's something biological behind the stress-free longevity claims, and it has to do with the telomeres and chromosomes in our DNA.

The 2009 Nobel Prize in Physiology/Medicine was awarded jointly to Elizabeth Blackburn, Carol Greider, and Jack Szostak for the discovery of how chromosomes are protected by telomeres and the enzyme telomerase.[8]

Essentially, they were recognized for discovering the molecular nature of telomeres, the ends of chromosomes that serve as protective caps essential for preserving genetic information, and for co-discovering telomerase, an enzyme that maintains telomere ends. Their work allowed us to understand the critical role telomeres and telomerase play in how we age.

DNA is the genetic material that provides the blueprint for who we are. Telomeres are the caps at the end of each strand of DNA that protect our chromosomes, like the plastic tips at the end of shoelaces. Without those tips, shoelaces become frayed until they can no longer do their job—just as, without telomeres, DNA strands become damaged to such an extent that our cells can't do their job. Telomeres get shorter each time a cell copies itself, but the important DNA stays intact. Eventually, telomeres get too short to do their job, causing our cells to age and stop functioning properly. Therefore, telomeres act as the aging clock in every cell.[9]

According to Blackburn, the enzyme telomerase adds bases to the ends of telomeres. In young cells, telomerase keeps telomeres from wearing down too much. But cells divide repeatedly during the course of our lives, and there is not enough telomerase to last forever, so the telomeres grow shorter and the cells age. Geneticist Richard Cawthon at the University of Utah found shorter telomeres are associated with shorter lives. Among people older than 60, those with shorter telomeres were three times more likely to die from heart disease and eight times more likely to die from infectious disease.[10]

Telomere length represents our biological age as opposed to our chronological age, and many of the behaviors associated with positive aging have the unintended effect of protecting and lengthening your telomeres. According to studies conducted by Blackburn and Epel, and Epel and Prather, there are a number of ways you can protect and lengthen your telomeres that are consistent with positive aging behavior.[11] These include: eating healthy foods, reducing stress, meditation, attitude, social interaction, and exercise. While it is clear that telomeres alone do not dictate life span, more interesting developments are sure to emerge on this fascinating front as an ever-increasing number of scientists continue to study telomeres and the benefits of stopping or possibly reversing the telomere shortening that happens as we age.

Final Thoughts

Why positive aging? The science supporting positive aging is tantalizing. The practice of positive aging is correlated to the length and health of our telomeres, which are directly related to aging. Positive aging likely lengthens life expectancy. Given the numerous benefits and life-changing effects of positive aging—which include enhanced physical, mental, emotional, and spiritual health, and an improved quality of life as you age—perhaps the more interesting question is, Why would anyone *not* practice positive aging?

So, now that the "Why" for practicing positive aging has been addressed, let's turn to the "How." What are the steps for practicing positive aging? My journey in battling cancer helped me stumble upon what I believe are the building blocks for practicing positive aging, which I will share with you throughout the rest of the book. Let's begin!

CHAPTER TWO

We Are in This Together

How many of us are aging, and how many of us are growing old? There is a difference.

Aging can be a wondrous journey, but your mindset will determine whether you find joy on this road. If you get anxious about physical decline and death, it will drive you mad and you will grow old quickly. But with the right approach, aging can become an adventure to treasure.

Aging can be a magnificent reality if you appreciate every moment in life, pursue a positive attitude, and adapt to physical and mental decline. Don't dwell on the marks of aging— if your knees break, use a walker; if your ears break, use a hearing aid. This is your encore, make the best of it. Staying alive is a wonderful concept but embracing life is a better one.

One of my most important lessons about aging came from a wise but very wet old man. I was seated comfortably in the lobby of my parents' senior living facility, waiting for a rainstorm to subside. I watched as a dark sky hurled sheets of rain onto the ground and against the window beside me, and then I saw an aged man with a walker drenched by the rain, moving unhurriedly toward the front entrance. I rushed outside and opened my umbrella above his head to shield him from the rain. He grimaced and said, "Get that umbrella away from me. Let me be!" I backed away and retreated into the building.

Minutes later, the elderly man approached me and said, "Son, I appreciate your act of kindness, but the rain against my skin felt wonderful to me. At my age, they are tears of joy."

What a revelation about growing old: Life is too short not to appreciate every moment. That man had learned a valuable lesson: Don't get hung up about getting wet when you can enjoy raindrops caressing your body.

As baby boomers reach their senior years, more and more of them are choosing to fill their lives with meaningful activities, postretirement employment, community service, and pleasurable experiences—like walking in the rain. I want to help spread these trends among the senior segment of our population.

Aging Rooms

I believe aging consists of two phases, which are discussed in more depth in chapter 10, Aging to the Other Side. In Phase I, we realize that we are aging and declining. Struggles and discomforts, such as hearing loss or arthritis, force us to face the harsh reality that our bodies will never be the same. In Phase II, we begin to recognize our own mortality. Any number of dire events, such as cancer or a severe heart attack, can open the curtains of finality.

However, our quality of life will be determined not by our stage of aging or by our physical or mental limitations, but by our choice of aging "rooms." We can choose to hang out in one of three places:

➢ The Positive Aging Room
➢ The Practical Aging Room
➢ God's Waiting Room

We want as many people as possible to hang out as often as possible in the Positive Aging Room, although most of us will spend some time in the Practical Aging Room. What we don't want to do is spend years moping around in God's Waiting Room.

The Positive Aging Room

The Positive Aging Room is like spending time in your home's family room. In most homes, the family room is where life happens. It's the most comfortable room in the house, the place you go to rest and recharge, to watch TV, play games, read books, and entertain friends. That's how your Positive Aging Room should feel, too. Positive aging means having the right attitude about growing old. It is about maintaining a healthy lifestyle and staying engaged fully in life, even as you experience physical and mental decline, so you don't lose a sense of control over your own life.

Plentiful research supports the benefits of positive aging (see the previous chapter). According to a study by Becca Levy (see chapter 15, Aging in America), senior citizens with positive self-perceptions of aging lived 7.5 years longer than those with negative self-perceptions of aging.[12]

My friend Sally practices positivity to the extreme. We can all learn from her example—I know I have. Sally doesn't believe in aging. Her objective is to escape the old mentality of aging and decline. She wants to grow younger and get healthier every day.

She knows that aging is a fact of life and time marches on as her physical body declines. But her philosophy is, "If we can imagine it, we can have it." She does not buy into society's perceptions of aging; she has opted out of aging. And she is not alone. There are an increasing number of baby boomers in this country, as well as Buddhists and Yogis and others, who do not introspectively think about aging and decline.

Sally tells me she is thinking about turning 35 on her next birthday. She says this will not be the first time she turned 35; it's happened several times over the past few years. She says 35 is a good year and she will stay there for some time.

Sally vibrates with positive energy, and lives a carefree, optimistic life. Yet in our reality, Sally is 82 years old and uses a walker for mobility and a hearing aid for listening to the rest of us complain about aging.

The Practical Aging Room

The Practical Aging Room is very much like your home's kitchen. Unless you *love* to cook, the kitchen is probably not your favorite room in the house. You spend time there because you need to keep yourself fed, but it's not the place you want to get trapped all day. There will be days on your aging journey that require a visit to the Practical Aging Room, but you don't want to get stuck here and never make it to the Positive Aging Room.

Most of us, in varying degrees, take a practical approach toward aging. We have not fully committed to embracing positivity but are hopeful that we will grow old gracefully. We stay positive about aging with a hint of anxiety and sometimes depression. We make the best of the situation while experiencing bouts of uneasiness and some loss of self-worth because we don't know how to find our way to the Positive Aging Room.

My mom and dad are in the Practical Aging Room. As of this writing, my mom is 89 and my dad is 96, and both deal with physical decline. My parents live in a senior living facility and walk gingerly with the aid of walkers. My mom has endured breast cancer, hip and shoulder surgery, diabetes, and hypertension, while my dad has endured an abdominal aortic aneurysm, significant hearing and vision loss, fluid in his lungs, and hypertension. My parents have dealt with their aging issues with dignity and vigor. But they also exhibited some emotional ups and downs as their physical and mental health declined. They are prime examples of practical aging: growing old gracefully.

Roberta also resides in the Practical Aging Room. Roberta is a wonderful woman, always complaining about life but with humor and sarcasm. She deserves to complain because she has endured a great deal of physical decline. Her knees have given out, so she uses a walker. She survived stage 2 lung cancer and heart valve replacement surgery. She knows her days are numbered yet focuses on living. She attends bingo every Wednesday at her church and visits with her grandchildren on Thursdays. She also paints beach and garden landscapes when she is physically up to it. Roberta resides in the Practical Aging Room because she remains anxious about growing old. She could easily find her way to the Positive Aging Room with a more positive mindset.

God's Waiting Room

People in God's Waiting Room do not embrace the power of positive aging, nor do they strive to grow old gracefully. They simply sit and wait for their name to be called, waiting to leave this life. People in God's Waiting Room are easy to spot. They show little energy or interest in the world around them. They are sometimes bitter and usually indifferent about their lives.

When you visit senior residential or care facilities, you can easily spot the people in God's Waiting Room. They are the ones who avoid social interaction and activities and feel there is little meaning left in life. They spend their days as if they are sitting in a laundromat waiting for clothes to dry. The dictionary says "to wait" means to stay in one place until someone comes for you. People in God's Waiting Room have lost their zest for life.

A Road Map to Positive Aging

My cancer opened my eyes to the fragility of life. It taught me how to cope with life-threatening disease, as well as the physical and mental decline that accompanies aging. I was diagnosed with stage 3 esophageal cancer when I was 62. My doctor made no promises, nor did he offer comforting words like "Don't worry, we'll beat this." Instead, he told me stage 3 esophageal cancer was life threatening as he laid out a game plan that began with six weeks of chemotherapy and radiation.

If that stage of the treatment proved to be successful, I would then need a seven-hour surgery on my esophagus and stomach. (An anatomy of my cancer battle is presented in Appendix D).

As I left the doctor's office, the nurse tried to reassure me about the future. "If you survive this," she said, "your cancer is an inconvenience." I didn't know at the moment, but she was so on-target.

I learned a great deal from my battle with cancer. In order to survive, I had little choice but to cope with the torturous effects of chemotherapy and radiation, and I had to learn to live with the fear that my cancer could spread (metastasize) and eventually kill me. I also had to learn to make post-surgery changes to my lifestyle. My stomach is now a long tube that runs up my chest; it is half the size of the original. Complications from my surgery require that I eat mostly soft foods (steak and pork chops are out) and liquids. I also must sleep on a 45-degree incline due to bile and acid reflux issues.

But I survived, and I now see cancer and its aftereffects as inconveniences. I have come to realize that every second, every minute, every day, every week, every month, every year, and every decade we are here in the physical realm we call life is a blessing.

My cancer journey is much like the aging journey. Every mark of aging, whether it is hearing loss, mobility loss, arthritis, Parkinson's disease, Alzheimer's disease, or multiple sclerosis, is an inconvenience. Inconvenience is something that causes trouble or problems. The inconveniences of aging are not life threatening—they are life changing. If you view the marks of aging as mere inconveniences, then the obstacles ahead, whatever they may be, aren't as intimidating.

This book aims to help you age successfully and gracefully by helping you cope with the inconveniences that come with a long shelf life. Allow it to serve as a road map to positive aging.

There is no dearth of advice about how to cope positively with life, aging, and suffering. The activities and practices presented in this book reflect bits and pieces taken from Buddhism, spiritualism, New Age beliefs, laws of attraction, mindfulness, and other notions and techniques that offer positive ways to deal with the suffering of aging.

Aging is a lifelong process, and physical and mental decline occurs throughout one's life span. With the right attitude and a healthy spirit, aging can bring about much joy and many rewards. Getting older is not all doom and gloom.

As individuals, we possess varying levels of physical, mental, and emotional strengths and weaknesses. The goal is to make adjustments in your life so you can better cope with "inconveniences," such as changes to your appearance, bodily functions, and mental health, and even life-threatening diseases.

During my battle with cancer, I discovered a number of practices and activities that helped me endure and recover. They are building blocks for a foundation for successful and positive aging. I introduce these six building blocks here and then investigate each more fully in the following chapters.

> ➤ Your inner spirit (the power of me)
> ➤ Mindfulness
> ➤ Positivity
> ➤ The Four A's
> ➤ Social support (the power of us)
> ➤ Balance

Your Inner Spirit (The Power of Me)

I believe we are more than our physical body—we also possess a spiritual body that is unaffected by time and aging. And I believe we need to spend more time on our spiritual side. We need to strengthen our spirit as our physical body declines. We need to go on a spiritual journey to prevent growing older.

In my view, nothing is more critical than a healthy spirit to cope with the marks of aging. This is the power of me. It is unfortunate, but most of us place little focus on our spirit as we live our lives. Most people are unaware of the powerful role that their spirits can play in their lives, particularly as they age.

Many religions and philosophies deal with this issue. Among them, as an example, is Buddhism, which is about finding freedom from suffering so humans can experience a peaceful existence. If your spirit effectively manages the suffering of aging, you allow joy into your life.

Whether you are an 18-year-old teenager, a 27-year-old woman about to be married, a 45-year-old businessman, a 67-year-old empty nester retiree, or a 91-year-old elderly woman, you will rely on your spirit to confront the struggles of aging. We feel the cumulative aches and pains in our back and other body parts with each passing year. We no longer jump as high or run as fast as in our younger years. Sexual drive peaks too soon for many of us. We take more and more meds to counter our physical and mental diminishment. Ultimately, many of us experience serious declines in quality of life or face life-threatening diseases. With the support of family and friends, combined with a healthy spirit, growing old can be a positive, if not exciting, journey.

Mindfulness

Mindfulness is living in the present moment, free from worries about the past or the future. This practice helps people appreciate every moment in life, an effective distraction from focusing on physical and mental decline.

Positivity

Learning to stay positive helps us maintain our self-worth as we face the challenges of aging. It helps us avoid negative thoughts and embrace life head-on.

The Four A's

Incorporating the Four A's—acceptance, adaptation, appreciation, attitude—into your life will help you find your way to the Positive Aging Room.

Social Support (The Power of Us)

Perhaps the greatest benefit of providing social support to a person experiencing the struggles of aging is to lift his or her spirit. One is a lonely number. We are all in this life together. If we help each other as we age, we can experience joy rather than suffering. This is the power of us.

Whether it is a life-threatening disease or a quality-of-life decline due to aging, people need support. You need other people who can act as your safety net.

I cannot overemphasize how important it is for humans to stick together as we age. Life can be wonderful in our senior years if we have a support network. Together we can make a difference.

MY JOURNEY

At 62 years old, cancer came a bit early from my perspective. You don't know how well you have it until you encounter a serious health crisis. No one knows better than me the importance of support from others when confronted with health issues, because I learned firsthand how family and friends can help you manage the suffering and lift your spirit.

My wife, family, and caring friends came through for me and gave me the emotional support, strength, and positivity I needed to get through the excruciating grind of cancer treatment. When I was nauseous, gagging on food, and vomiting from the cumulative effects of the poisonous chemotherapy, my wife was by my side to help me. My family surrounded me with an endless amount of love while my friends volunteered to help with weekly household chores.

My support network literally saved my life during my battle with cancer. Nobody lives in isolation; life is a group outing.

Balance

Finding the right balance in your life as you age is critical to successful aging. The challenge is that we become increasingly out of balance as we age. Aging leaves many of us feeling unsettled, anxious, and confused about who we are. Life balancing includes making adjustments to your lifestyle, social interactions, priorities, and expectations.

United We Age

Conventional wisdom says older people should retire, shrivel up, and fade into the sunset. We live in a youth-dominated society with heavy doses of celebrity worship and the persistent message that old is not cool. Older people are relegated to the backside of society. Conventional wisdom needs to be turned inside out and on its head, and I hope that this book can help change the way our society views aging while also changing the way we age.

Parents and educators teach children how to be firemen, lawyers, doctors, teachers, and construction workers, but no one teaches us how to be 70, 80, or 90 years old. No one teaches us how to deal with life-threatening diseases or wrinkles, failing eyesight, deteriorating mobility, and memory loss. We don't know how to grow old, and we don't know how to treat the elderly in our society.

In some cultures, senior citizens are not cast aside. In China, young people are expected to defer to older people, let them speak first, sit only after their elders are seated, and not contradict them. In some African communities, older citizens command great respect. But as China and other senior-friendly societies become modernized, cultural norms—including honoring elders—wither away.

We live in a youth-obsessed nation where aging is out and being young is in. Young celebrities like Kim Kardashian are revered, while the elderly are put out to pasture. People spend billions of dollars on antiaging creams and surgical procedures to eliminate wrinkles because wrinkles make them look old. What if we viewed wrinkled faces as reflections of life's experiences that took years to create?

Many older people are ashamed or embarrassed to display marks of aging in our forever-young society because they fear being labeled frail and useless. Wrinkles are ugly, wheelchairs represent helplessness, and hearing aids reflect weakness. The cultural belief that aging equals decline and poor health has created self-fulfilling prophecies as seniors surrender to infirmities and sink into depression, believing their usefulness is gone.

Others fight to stay relevant with antiaging products and current fashion. There is nothing inherently wrong with wanting to appear young if it makes you feel good, raises your confidence, and promotes a healthier lifestyle. The problem comes when you buy into the societal messaging that staying young is superior to growing old.

My hope is to inspire Americans to unite as we age. There are literally millions of senior citizens living alone in America today experiencing quality-of-life decline with no support network. Without social support, they are having a difficult time coping. Quality of life and life expectancy decline for people lacking a social support network (e.g., spouse, family, friends).

We need local networks of support across America for people with life-threatening diseases/conditions and for people experiencing quality-of-life decline due to aging, especially for people living alone. These networks can bring together people of all ages to lift the spirits and enhance the quality of life for aging people across the country.

Our Western ways continue to promote forever-young attitudes that ignore the spirituality, wisdom, and creativity of older adults. Older people need to feel relevant, respected, and useful if they are to live meaningful lives with dignity. Their lives need to be celebrated, not marginalized. People need to support each other as they confront the marks of aging. It would be commendable if people of all generations joined (figuratively or literally) a united we age movement to offer the emotional support necessary to make a difference in an older person's life.

A Journey of Inconvenience

From a positive aging perspective, cancer is an inconvenience of aging, and so is every other mark of aging. They are inconveniences because life is precious at all ages and in all stages—not just when we are young and healthy and strong. We live on this Earth and we die on this Earth, so while we are living every moment is precious. That is why we live in the moment. As long as we can smell the roses and hear the ocean waves hit the shoreline, we have a quality of life worth savoring.

The remainder of this book serves as a guide that will, hopefully, place you on the wondrous journey of positive aging. This book will help you tap into your spirit, seek and find social support, and practice any combination of mindfulness, positivity, the Four A's, and balance as you confront the inconveniences of aging. I've learned we are not at war with Father Time; we never have been. We are only battling ourselves when we resist the natural process of aging. Aging is God's (or the universe's) way of telling us it's time to transition to the other side. From a spiritual perspective, it's the beginning of a new journey.

Writing this book has been profoundly therapeutic. I had a difficult time coping with cancer at 62 years old; I became bitter about my diagnosis and developed a heightened fear of finality. But my social network lifted my spirit, and, in turn, my spirit rediscovered a passion for living. Although my post-cancer self is physically weaker than my pre-cancer self, I am spiritually stronger than I've ever been before. My journey has taken a different path today, and it is a more robust and satisfying path. I now have a positive aging attitude, and I want to help you find and maintain your own positive aging attitude while also encouraging our society to recognize the worth of aging.

Hopefully, "We are in this together" will become a mantra for all of us.

CHAPTER THREE

The Power of Me: Inner Spirit

If we imagine the practice of positive aging as an orchestra playing beautiful music, our inner spirit is the conductor.

A story I love is about a poor panhandler sitting on an old storage trunk begging for money. A wealthy man dressed in a dapper suit stopped to give him a few dollars and asked, "How long have you been sitting on this trunk soliciting for money?" The beggar answered, "I've been sitting on this old trunk for over three years. This is a pretty good street corner; some days I do well and some days I go hungry."

"Have you ever opened the trunk to see what's inside?" the man asked.

"No, I never thought to open it; it's locked," the beggar replied.

The man put down his briefcase and picked up a rock and pounded on the trunk's lock until it broke. The beggar opened the trunk to find a treasure of gold. He had not known how wealthy he was until he looked inside.

Just as there was treasure inside that trunk, even though the beggar didn't realize it, there is something extraordinary inside all of us. Some call it a spirit, others call it a soul. I will refer to it as our spirit. One of the keys to effectively manage age-related decline is to rely on a social network of support, which in turn lifts the spirit. A healthy spirit is a critical ingredient to successful aging. As you experience physical and mental decline with aging, focus on strengthening your spirit; the spirit is not affected by the marks of aging.

Your spirit is your best friend. It is part of your social support group—it is the power of me. As humans age, the physical body declines while the spiritual body continues to grow. I believe aging is about your spirit taking center stage—and I'm not alone in this belief. Spiritual awareness is on the rise in America. Meditation groups and yoga classes are becoming increasingly popular across the nation, with some companies offering meditation to their employees. More and more people use phrases like "universal life energy" and "unity consciousness," which reflect the beliefs that there is a consciousness connecting all life. The revolution of the spirit is here.

Follow your spirit and the marks of aging become inconveniences rather than burdens. They are inconveniences because they do not threaten your life itself; they only threaten your way of life and possibly the quality of your life.

Embrace your spirit and you will perceive aging through a stronger lens with greater clarity. You will be more confident and secure, and you will no longer be embarrassed or ashamed about the marks of aging you may bear, whether they are from battling cancer or heart disease, a decline in physical appearance, a disabled body function, or a mental impairment. The goal is to have a healthier and longer life span filled with meaning.

To my knowledge, there is no scientific evidence as of yet supporting the notion of a spirit or soul. Nevertheless, an overwhelming majority of humans on this planet believe they possess a spirit or soul. I'm one of them. Most traditional Judeo-Christian religions believe in an afterlife where the spirit/soul transcends to Heaven, while many Eastern religions (e.g., Buddhism) believe the spirit/soul reincarnates to relive in future physical bodies. The common thread among these beliefs is that most humans believe they are more than just their physical body—they believe they possess a spirit/soul, and the physical body serves as a vessel for the spirit to exist in the physical realm.

According to the 2014 General Social Survey, led by psychologist Jean Twenge of San Diego State University, fewer Americans say they believe in God or pray regularly—yet more people believe in an afterlife, nonetheless. The study surveyed 58,000 people and found that 80 percent of Americans said they believe in an afterlife, up from 73 percent in 1972.[13]

If this is so, shouldn't we focus more of our energies as we age on growing and strengthening our spirits rather than focusing on the decline and decay of our physical bodies? It is your spirit that defines you, not your physical appearance.

But try telling that to any teenager getting ready for a Saturday-night date. Or for that matter, try telling it to any woman who is putting on a nice outfit, applying makeup, and fixing her hair to run to the grocery store to pick up some lettuce and milk. The importance of physical appearance is firmly entrenched in American society. Most people are more focused on how they appear to be—both physically and socially—than how they really are. Many of us care more about how other people perceive us than how we genuinely feel about ourselves.

Not surprisingly, superficial appearances matter less as we grow older. Older people covered in wrinkles and age spots become more focused on their health and the authenticity of relationships than with physical attributes and social status.

Interest in spirituality and aging has risen during this past decade due in part to growing evidence that spiritual and religious practices generate positive physical and mental health outcomes. We are enjoying longer life spans today, and this reality highlights the importance of spirituality in older people to better cope with the potentially lengthy process of aging. Fortunately, studies have shown that people become more spiritual with age.

Spirituality makes it easier to maintain a positive attitude when experiencing physical and mental decline, which is why it is the first of the six building blocks in the Power of Positive Aging program. It takes discipline to do the right thing when everything seems to be against you. How can you be emotionally strong when you are emotionally drained?

Exploring Your Spirit

It is generally acknowledged that humans are composed of body, mind, and spirit (or soul). However, there is little consensus among cognitive scientists, philosophers, and religious scholars about the spirit's functions and its relationship with the mind. Let's explore some of the more prominent explanations, so we can better understand how spirit is linked to positive aging.

Scientific Explanations

The mind is a set of cognitive faculties that enables consciousness, perception, thinking, judgment, feeling, and memory. Over the decades, there have been numerous attempts to develop an understanding of the nature of the mind and its relation to the brain and nervous system.

In the psychiatric field, the computational theory claims that the mind is separate from physical existence. This theory asserts that the nervous system is an information processing system that works by translating changes in the body and the environment into a language of neural impulses that represent the animal–environment relationship. The computational theory allows people to conceptually separate the mind from the brain and body. We can conceive of the mind as the flow of information through the nervous system and this flow of information can be conceptually separated from the biophysical matter that makes up the nervous system. To better illustrate this concept, scientists use the analogy of a book. The book's physical characteristics can be considered as roughly akin to the brain. However, the information content (i.e., the story the book tells or the information it conveys) is akin to the mind. The mind, then, is the information instantiated in and processed by the nervous system. Therefore, we can conceptually separate the mind from the brain, which may help us conceptually separate the spirit from our body.

Religious/Supernatural Traditions and Explanations

According to Buddhism, the mind has two fundamental qualities: clarity and knowing. Clarity refers to the fact that the mind has no physical characteristics, while knowing refers to the mind functioning to cognize or perceive objects. The mind is aware of the contents of experience, so in order to exist, the mind must be cognizing an object. There is also an intimate connection between the mind and perception. A person's state of mind plays a crucial role in his or her experiences of happiness and suffering; this is crucial in the context of aging.

Buddhists believe in the intimate relationships between mind and body and in the existence of physiological centers within the body. Physical yoga exercises and meditation techniques aimed at training the mind can have positive effects on health and thus enhance the aging process. Further, there are some meditation techniques that make it possible to separate your mind from your physical body.

Many people believe the spirit/soul is part of the "upper mind," which suggests that part of the mind is not attached to the physical body. Many Buddhists and New Age enthusiasts assert that the purpose of meditation is to clear the mind, so you can tap into your spirit/soul.

Traditional religion makes a distinction between a spirit and soul. The spirit is the element in humanity that gives us the ability to have an intimate relationship with God. Spirit refers to the immaterial part of humanity that "connects" with God (John 4:24). The soul is the essence of humanity's being; it is who we are.

Spirituality comes in many shapes and sizes. People involved in New Age spirituality proclaim that they are spiritual but not religious. They are aware of a connection or relationship with something that goes beyond sensory perceptions. Religious people make the connection between spirit and God. The broadest definition is that spirituality is the affirmation of something beyond the physical realm that relates God or a universal entity to a community of people and connects them with a nurturing wholeness.

My Explanations

I make no distinction between a spirit and a soul. I make no claims about which beliefs are true and which are false. To me, all beliefs are possibilities, and eventually science will uncover the truths about life, the universe, whether spirits and souls exist, and if there is after-life. For the purposes of this book, religious and spiritual proclivities are unimportant, as is the difference between a belief in God as the almighty or God as a universal energy source.

The only assumption I make is that when we pass on, our physical bodies are left behind and our spirits transcend. Focus on growing your spirit while your body is decaying, and you will age gracefully.

Tap into Your Spirit

So, how do you nurture and grow your spirit? As you rely on your five senses (sight, hearing, touch, taste, smell) to nurture your physical body, you should rely on your intuitive perception to nurture your spirit.

Seek out moments that allow your spirit to reveal itself. Create more of these moments as you encounter the marks of aging, and you will feel that sense of calm and infinite peace in your inner self. Harness it; capture the feeling and call upon it often as you age.

How do you create these spiritually nourishing moments? Engage in activities that make it easy and fun to tap into your spirit. You can reach your spirit by clearing your mind through meditation and other spirit-related activities that can be inserted seamlessly into your daily routines.

Just as you exercise your physical body to gain strength and stay healthy and fit, your brain/mind also needs to be exercised so you can tap into your spirit. Someone who has never trained for running would have a difficult time finishing a 26-mile marathon, but with proper training running a marathon is an attainable goal. Similarly, someone who has never trained in a spiritual sense may experience initial frustration but in due time will likely succeed.

To get started, here are some popular ways that people tap into their inner spirit. I used some of these during my battle with cancer.

Tame Your Ego

An untamed ego is your spirit's greatest enemy. Not surprisingly, your ego responds negatively to overall decline in physical appearance, as well as to decline in bodily functions (e.g., digestive problems). I liken it to a jealous 6-year old boy trying to gain the attention of his parents over his 3-year old sister—the ego steps in front of the spirit at every opportunity. Taming your ego is a mandatory first step in tapping into your spirit, and it comes before employing the other steps for coping with aging.

You begin by becoming aware that your ego heavily influences your thoughts and actions and that your ego makes it more difficult to age gracefully. Then you will realize that *you* are in control of your thoughts, not your ego. Do not rush the process; your objective is to make a little progress each day at taming your ego.

Hold a picture of your younger self up to the mirror and contrast it to the person you see now. Your ego will long to be young again and might emit a series of emotions like sadness, anger, resentment, and shame.

Take note of everything old about you (e.g., wrinkles, age spots, hair loss), and then just say no to your ego. Instead, view your physical marks of aging as a badge of honor. Feel a sense of pride in reaching this point in your life. Tell your ego that growing old is a good thing; it's something to be proud of.

MY JOURNEY

During my battle with cancer, I discovered a number of ways to lift my spirit while coping with chemotherapy and radiation treatments, as well as when I was dealing with the anguish involved with the pre- and post-surgery periods.

When first diagnosed with cancer, it was my ego that had a difficult time. My ego was bruised and unable to accept that I had cancer. Other people got cancer, not me. I had to push my ego aside and accept my fate. This was the first step in coping with and battling cancer.

Perhaps you have experienced times when your spirit unexpectedly surged ahead of your ego. For me, one such time occurred when I vacationed in Costa Rica years ago. I was walking in a place where the rain forest meets the ocean. As I strolled on the white sands of the Costa Rican beach, to my left was a breathtaking sight of clear blue ocean waves hitting against the shore, while to my right was a picturesque view of a tropical rain forest—with monkeys jumping from tree to tree and exotic birds boasting the colors of the rainbow perched on tree limbs. In that moment, I was free of past and future thoughts. I felt no anxiety or sadness. I felt happiness and joy and I didn't have a care in the world.

My spirit had come for a visit and, for a while at least, displaced my attention-seeking ego.

Seek Peaceful Moments

At least two or three times per day, put yourself in a place where you can be "far from the madding crowd" and away from all distractions. This could be in your bedroom, or outside on a back porch, or during a walk in the park. The objective is to capture some moments where you can find peace of mind. These moments better prepare you to summon your spirit.

During my six-week chemotherapy/radiation treatment in Tampa, Florida, I would take long walks at the Residence Inn where I was staying. I found a path that was lined with tall trees that had a calming effect on me. This was my time of reflection, and my spirit led the way.

Walking puts your mind in a relaxed state of clear thought. Walking gives your brain a chance to wander and free itself from any troubling thoughts, which is a prerequisite for tapping into your spirit. I know I'm tapping into my spirit when I walk alone and think.

Meditate

Meditation is a practice that promotes relaxation, builds internal energy (or life-force), and develops compassion, love, kindness, and an overall sense of well-being. It is perhaps the most effective practice of spirituality. Meditation involves focusing on an object, a point in space, or a mantra (in Buddhist or yoga practices). Some physicians and health centers now routinely recommend meditation or yoga and include them as part of integrated health programs. See detailed instructions for meditation in chapter 4, Mindfulness.

Facilitate an Out-of-Body Experience

Have you ever experienced an out-of-body experience? Over 25 percent of adults in the United States claim to have experienced at least one out-of-body experience.

An out-of-body experience, or OBE, is an experience that typically involves a sensation of floating outside one's body or, in some cases, the feeling of perceiving one's physical body as if from a place outside one's body. People who have experienced an OBE tend to hold a strong belief that their spirit is separate from their physical body.

OBEs can be induced by deep meditation, sounds that stimulate the brain, and near-death experiences, among others. However, not everyone believes in the validity of OBEs. Neuroscientists and psychologists regard OBEs as dissociative experiences arising from different psychological and neurological factors.

Some people take OBEs a step further than just believing that their spirit can separate from their physical body. Some believe that once they have an OBE and their spirit leaves their physical body, they have acquired the skills for their spirit to travel in the astral plane. The astral plane refers to other dimensions in the universe that some call the heavens.

Whether astral travel is an illusion of the mind or real is way outside the scope of this book. Our purpose is to provide another piece of information that leads to the belief that we humans are more than our physical bodies.

So, how do you conduct an out-of-body experience? Robert Monroe's 1971 book *Journeys Out of the Body* demonstrated how audio technology could facilitate OBEs. Monroe conducted research on human consciousness from which he produced evidence that specific sound patterns have identifiable effects on our states of consciousness. By testing certain combinations of frequencies on himself, Monroe was able to encounter what he termed an out-of-body experience. Monroe went on to develop Hemi Sync, an audio technology that facilitates OBEs. Just Google "Hemi Sync" and you will be able to purchase his audio CDs of sounds.

You may be thinking this is all far-fetched, but I've actually experienced an out-of-body experience on multiple occasions. Whether this was really my spirit rising out of my body or just an illusion based on psychological or neurological factors, I cannot say.

In any event, here is how I experienced an OBE using the Monroe Hemi Sync method:

➢ Lie in bed with hands at your side and get as comfortable as you can. You need to place yourself in the best position and environment to achieve success. You should be in a distraction-free environment where you can darken the room and remain undisturbed during the 30- to 45-minute exercise. Loosen any tight clothing and remove shoes and glasses (or contacts).

➢ You will hear a voice on the Hemi Sync CD and then you will hear sounds. There are three steps that you must follow for any OBE exercise: create an energy conversion box; recite the affirmation; and conduct resonant tuning.

➢ An energy conversion box is symbolic of a location where you can place all your worries and concerns, leaving you free and unencumbered. Create it in your mind, even if you don't see, hear, or feel it.

➢ Say the affirmation: "I am more than my physical body." The affirmation helps you focus your attention on what you want to accomplish during the exercise. It helps you focus your intent, thereby enabling you to become more aware of your expanding consciousness.

➢ The final step is resonant tuning, which is a breathing exercise to help you vitalize and charge your entire system. It promotes an accelerated gathering of your vibrational energy while reducing your internal dialogue. From the Monroe CD you will hear strange, eerie sounds of a symphonic or synthesized nature. You need to put your mind into the rhythmic sound waves.

➢ If you are successful (and it may take three to ten exercises to get there), you will feel a tingling sensation throughout your body. When you do, keep your mind focused and soon the tingling will change to vibrations, which will get more intense by the second, capturing your entire body, head to toe.

➢ And then it could happen—you will be looking down at your body. You will have experienced an OBE. It is possible that you will have a sensation that your spirit is floating freely and drifting upward toward the bedroom ceiling. It will be a glorious feeling.

When it is over, you will say to yourself, *Did this just happen, or was this a dream? Was this my imagination, or reality?* Personally, I don't know whether to believe or not to believe, but I'm glad for the experience. In any event, these Hemi Sync sounds will take you on a spiritual journey whether you experienced an OBE or not. And you will certainly have the sensation that you are more than your physical body, an important tenet for the practice of positive aging.

Connect Through Crystals

There is a small but growing segment of people in America today who utilize crystals as an aid to awaken their spirits. Crystals have had prominence in ancient rituals and practices over the past millennium. For believers, humans emit an energy into the universe, and crystals absorb energy vibrations emitted from their surroundings and then send them back into the world. People connect with crystals and feed off their emission of positive energy, lifting their vibrations and moving them to a spiritual state.

Crystals are physical forms of the Earth's energy. When you connect with your crystal, your crystal gets to know you, in a sense, based on your vibration. It is believed that programming your crystals with specific intentions creates a special aura in your environment, helping you fight off any negativity that may be affecting your well-being. This is particularly useful for people seeking to tap their spirit and embrace positivity as they age.

The question of whether the power of crystals is real is up to each one of us. For purposes of tapping our spirit, believers should use crystals as an aid. For nonbelievers, there may still be a positive psychological effect of using crystals, thinking that *maybe* they have the power to tap into your spirit.

If you acquire a crystal, put it into practice by wearing it as jewelry, placing it in your home, or carrying it in your pocket. Here are five crystals associated with facilitating a spiritual journey:

Clear Quartz. Quartz is one of the most basic crystals to begin your spiritual journey with. Quartz carries the power to cleanse your thoughts and clear your mind. Once you feel connected to your quartz, clarify your intentions for the stone and trust that it is listening.

Selenite. This stone is known for unblocking stagnant energies, ensuring a positive flow of vibrations between you and your crystal. Selenite is one of the most powerful tools for removing negativity as you age.

Shungite. This stone contains natural antioxidants, making it a powerful healer of health-hazardous energies to the body. It can be used for detoxification and relief from anxiety as you age.

Amethyst. It is believed that this stone acts as an energetic shield containing a spiritual light around your body. This stone is particularly useful for people confronting physical and mental decline because it helps strengthen your spiritual body, as well as boosting your self-worth.

Citrine. This stone carries the energy of the sun and promotes happiness and positivity as we cope with the marks of aging. Citrine is a useful crystal for people as they age because it fills you with optimism and motivates you to form good habits for achieving balance in your life.

Pray

Prayer is a profound way to tap into your spirit and communicate with what some believe to be godlike powers or a higher self. For many, prayer is an effective form of coping that helps older people as they physically and mentally age.

I did not lean on prayer during my battle with cancer. I guess I felt awkward communicating with something I'm not sure about. However, nearly 60 percent of Americans report praying daily. Interestingly, group prayer is associated with a greater well-being and happiness, while solitary prayer is associated with depression and loneliness. There is some scientific validation of the benefits of prayer, in terms of health outcomes, but it is not conclusive. Critics of prayer maintain that any perceived benefits of prayer are likely due to a placebo effect. However, until science proves otherwise, prayer is an effective way to summon our spirit and is useful for anyone dealing with the marks of aging or a life-threatening disease.

Practice Yoga

Sometimes it is necessary to prepare your body for meditation by stretching and building strength. Yoga, an ancient Indian health regimen, is a practice that accomplishes this task by creating balance in the body's energy centers through developing both strength and flexibility. Yoga unites the body, mind, and spirit, and teaches your body how to tap into your spirit. It helps to discipline your mind, and it trains your nervous system so it's easier for you to process spiritual energy. Another benefit of yoga is that it can be used in combination with other treatments for anxiety, stress, depression, and other mental disorders.

While I've personally only dabbled in yoga, many of my friends and acquaintances have benefited greatly from it. Yoga classes are plentiful in every community. It will be well worth your time.

Stimulate Your Mind

Your mind is the gateway to your spirit, so conditioning and stimulating it are essential for achieving your spiritual journey. There are numerous ways to prepare your mind for a spiritual journey. I've selected the ways that I believe are practical for aging boomers and senior citizens to implement.

Drawing. Drawing or painting stimulates the right side of the brain, which inspires creativity. The more creative you are, the more you are in touch with your spirit. I don't draw because I can't even draw a straight line, but if you have any artistic talent or interest, painting and drawing are wonderful ways to stimulate your mind and touch your spirit. In fact, art therapy has become a popular activity for older people in assisted living facilities. It is particularly beneficial for people in memory care facilities who are afflicted with dementia.

Music. Studies have demonstrated that musical sounds strengthen the right side of the brain. Listening to music is a mentally healthy activity that can take you into a meditative state.

I've observed the positive effects of music on senior citizens at my parents' senior living community. Every Friday night is music night, and a semiprofessional entertainer sings songs from the 1940s, 50s, and 60s to an audience composed of 70-, 80-, and 90-year-olds. The first time I attended one of these sessions I was astounded at the mesmerizing effect that the sweet sounds and familiar lyrics of the music had on most of the seniors in the audience. It was like the music touched their souls and spirits, and for 60 minutes their lives achieved peace and harmony.

My 96-year old dad listens to classical music to escape the realities of life and aging, whereas Bruce Springsteen songs do it for me.

Writing. When you write, you strengthen your brain's natural ability to convey thoughts and feelings. Writing journals, diaries, blog entries, and stories are excellent ways to fulfill the needs of your brain. For older people, writing a bio legacy (your life story) can be an effective way to tap into your spirit while also adding meaning to your life.

For me, writing this book was a home run—the most stimulating activity I've ever been involved in.

Mind Games. Mind games are thought-provoking and challenging activities. Participating in games such as crossword puzzles, sudoku, chess, or card games is mentally stimulating and tends to engage both the left and right sides of the brain. If you are retired, dedicate a specific period of time each day (say, 3:00 p.m.) to participate in a mind game. Card games like gin, poker, and bridge are popular at most senior centers.

Reading. Reading is exercise for the mind. It would be beneficial to do some form of reading every day, and there are plenty of sources to choose from: books, magazines, newspapers, or news websites.

Love Yourself

For me, love derives from the spirit, not the ego. The more you love yourself (self-love), the closer you are to your spirit. As we age, some of us feel a diminished sense of self-worth and some may wallow in self-pity. Never doubt how truly awesome you are. You deserve love—and lots of it—from yourself. And as soon as you can give yourself more love, you are much closer to tapping into the energy within your higher self.

Final Thoughts

There is a magic wand for dealing with the inconveniences of aging—our spirit. I've come to believe that embracing and connecting with your spirit is a monumental event in life that opens a whole new world filled with wonderful possibilities. There is no better prescription for aging (or battling a challenging disease) than tapping into your spirit. Tapping into my spirit was without a doubt my greatest asset during my battle with cancer.

When you are down and drowning in past thoughts or negativity, people will tell you that you need to live in the present and feel the touch of God. I believe this advice is on target, whether you are a religious person or not. (If you are not religious, just substitute "spirit" for God.) Touch your spirit and you will be set free.

CHAPTER FOUR

Mindfulness

One of the secrets to successful positive aging is to live in the present moment. We mustn't worry about the future or dwell in the past when confronting physical and mental decline. For many people, growing old means a simpler way of life filled with fewer distractions. This may make it easier to live in the present than when we were young and occupied with so many family, social, and work responsibilities.

Choosing to live in the past or worry about the future is self-defeating for older people because it robs them of the chance to truly live. The only important moment is the present moment. This should be quite clear to older people, whose best interest is to appreciate every precious moment in life. It is especially clear to people experiencing life-threatening diseases/conditions.

Mindfulness has enjoyed a surge in popularity in the past two decades, as reflected both in the media and in psychotherapy practices, and also in the habits and practices of millions of ordinary people. *Mindfulness* means living in the moment and awakening to experience. For our purposes, mindfulness is important because it creates the right mindset for successfully aging.

Mindfulness is closely associated with Buddhist meditative practices and can be developed using the meditation techniques presented in this chapter. Meditation is typically practiced sitting or lying in a comfortable position as you focus on breathing in and out. By focusing your awareness on your breathing, you empty your mind of other thoughts. If you become distracted and a stray thought pops into your mind (which *will* happen from time to time), accept the distraction in a nonjudgmental way and then focus again on breathing.

Mindfulness is realizing that you are not your mind. You are not all those thoughts, judgments, and noise running through your head. You are the awareness of your mind's activities; you are just "awareness"— you are at peace.

To attain true mindfulness, you should aspire to 30-minute meditation sessions. But you'll need to build yourself up to that level—the more you meditate, the easier it becomes to maintain awareness of your breathing and achieve peace of mind.

It may surprise many Westerners who are unfamiliar with Buddhism, but one of Buddhism's primary missions is to deal with aging and finality, in which mindfulness plays an important role. Buddhism was founded by a man pursuing freedom from suffering caused by sickness, aging, and death. Therefore, Buddhism provides a path to follow in dealing with the inconveniences of aging.

To gain a deeper appreciation for today's Buddhism and how it helps us deal with aging, here is how the Buddha achieved nirvana and spread his teachings.

The Buddha and His Teachings

Prince Siddhartha sat down to meditate under a large bodhi tree, facing east. He promised himself, "I will not give up until I achieve my goal to find freedom from suffering, for myself and all people."

Siddhartha fell into a deep meditation. He let go of all outside disturbances and emptied his mind of all past pleasures and thoughts. Within the stillness of his mind, he focused on discovering the truth about life and suffering. His mind embarked on a journey through his previous lives.

Siddhartha saw how beings are reborn according to the law of cause and effect, or karma. He saw that doing good things resulted in peace, not suffering. He realized that suffering came from greed and greed came from believing that we are more important than everybody else.

Siddhartha's ultimate journey was achieving nirvana, a state of mind that was free from any suffering. So, at the age of 35, Siddhartha became the Buddha, the Supreme Enlightened One.

The Buddha set out to teach ideal truths (dharma) to his people. He taught the other monks the truth about life and suffering and showed them how to end suffering by achieving enlightenment.

The Buddha taught the Four Noble Truths. The first Noble Truth was that suffering exists; the second was about the cause of suffering; the third was that it is possible to end suffering; and the fourth explained the path to ending suffering.

The Buddha also taught the Five Precepts, which were training rules to create good karma: Respect and be kind to all living things. Do not kill or steal. Do not be unfaithful to your wife. Do not lie. And do not take intoxicants. The Buddha stressed that there is a cause for everything and whatever comes into existence will also decay.

The Buddha told his disciples to practice and teach these basic principles. In simple terms, Buddha's message was: Do good things and purify your mind.

Today's Mindfulness Teachings

Many people in modern society have taken the baton from Buddha—Eckhart Tolle is one of them. Tolle wrote a best-selling book, *The Power of Now*, promulgating the virtues of living in the present. In this spiritual classic, Tolle reveals how he experienced a state of desperation when he hit rock bottom in his life. To quote Tolle:

"I could feel that a deep longing for non-existence was becoming much stronger than my desire to continue to live."

Then, as Tolle tells us, his mind stopped—there were no more thoughts. He sensed an energy force and his body began to shake. He heard the words, "resist nothing," and suddenly, he felt no fear. Ever since, Tolle has lived in the moment, in a state of peace and bliss, and he has dedicated his life to helping others do the same.

What does the act of mindfulness actually do for us as we age?

MY JOURNEY

For me personally, mindfulness is—everything. Before my cancer diagnosis at 62, I had a difficult few years. In my mid-50s, I was a casualty of the financial crisis. I was the chief economist of the nation's largest trade association, the National Association of Realtors, and I was riding high during the real estate boom. I had media appearances (television, print, radio, Internet) and gave speeches across the nation. I authored a book (*Are You Missing the Real Estate Boom?*), in which I projected that the boom would continue for another two to three years. However, the real estate boom turned into a real estate bust just as my book was released. I was flooded with negative publicity and vilified on the Internet. Reporters and bloggers believed I had misled people into buying homes that would soon turn into foreclosures. No one bothered to learn that I followed my own advice and invested my money in real estate. I truly believed the boom would continue and I bet on my beliefs by acquiring seven investment properties during that time period.

I was in a sorrowful place—my world had turned upside down and inside out. My mind flooded with thoughts of nonexistence. For the next several years I was depressed about my past and frightened about my future. It was only when I learned to live in the present (through meditation and other techniques) that I was able to "right" my life. When I decided to let go of the past and not to worry about things that haven't happened yet, I experienced a paradigm shift in consciousness. My self-worth, which had hit bottom, gained an upward trajectory.

Living in the present moment is how I survived my personal crisis. It is how I survived cancer, and it will be how I survive and cope with growing old. Living in the present moment means I know what's happening in the here and now. For example, if I raise my hand, I am conscious of the fact that I'm raising my hand. My mind is lifting my arm toward the ceiling and my fingers extend outward, waving toward the ceiling. I am not distracted by any other thoughts.

For me, the beauty of meditation is that after I meditate for a few minutes, I have the sensation that I am more than just my physical body. This broadened mindset has become a psychological advantage that I want to have as I continue to experience physical decline with aging.

To be mindful means being aware, and to be aware in the present moment takes concentration and energy. Reflections of past events and worries and anxiety about the future are always there, ready to distract you. You can acknowledge them, but then shift focus and return to the present moment.

Ways to Live in the Present

Aging generally promises a simpler life, which creates an opportunity to live in the present.

If you feel negativity about your older self, you are likely thinking about the past, reflecting on what it was like to be younger looking, free of wrinkles, etc. Practice living in the present and you will minimize thoughts about your younger self. If you have nothing to compare your older appearance to, there is no benchmark—and thus there is no reason for negativity.

Spending time with nature is one way I enjoy living in the present. I find time to take long walks outside in my neighborhood. You would be surprised how a walk by yourself helps you be more in the moment. I also practice simple meditation of just 5 minutes in the morning and at night. If you can practice simple meditation on a regular basis (say, every Wednesday, Friday, and Sunday), you will live a more mindful existence.

Here are some ways that people today live in the present.

Meditate

Of course, the most effective way to achieve mindfulness is to practice intense meditative techniques. As mentioned earlier, to attain true mindfulness you should aspire to 30-minute meditation sessions. The more you meditate, the easier it becomes to maintain awareness of your breathing, which helps empty the mind.

Here is a simple way to meditate:

> ➢ Sit or lie comfortably
> ➢ Close your eyes
> ➢ Breathe naturally
> ➢ Focus your attention on your breathing and how your body moves with each inhalation and exhalation
> ➢ Focus and repeat a mantra such as "ohm" or "I'm"
> ➢ Come back into focus when you wander
> ➢ You are now in a meditative state

I admit, I had a difficult time meditating during my treatment; I was easily distracted due to my heightened anxiety. However, instead of getting frustrated and more anxious because of failed meditation, I chose to practice what I call simple meditation—meditating for just 2 to 5 minutes per session. Although meditating for less than 5 minutes seemed fruitless, it was effective over a period. Of course, if you can meditate for 30 minutes or more, do it.

After meditating, people are more likely to focus their attention in the present. Meditation makes your mind calmer and more focused. Even a simple 2-to-5-minute breathing meditation can help you overcome the stress of aging, and it will help you find a measure of inner peace and balance. If you are able to perform an intense 30-minute meditation, you will transform negative energy to positive energy, and go from being despondent to satisfied. Ripening positive thoughts is the purpose of the transforming meditations found in the Buddhist tradition.

When you achieve a deep meditative state, I believe you touch your spirit. You will experience a calming sensation; you will feel less stress and you will be free from your ego. Thoughts about the past and worries about the future are absent; you are now in the present moment. Meditating several times a day is like refueling your spiritual tank—it gives you the spiritual energy to cope with the inconveniences of aging on a daily basis.

For people who do not want to fully integrate meditation into their lives, I suggest trying out my simple approach of meditating two times per day for just 2 to 5 minutes for each session. Apps such as Simple Habit, Calm, and Headspace offer brief, easy-to-use meditation sessions. (See chapter 14, A Lifestyle Plan for Positive Aging, for additional suggestions.)

Morning. Take 2 to 5 minutes out of your morning to meditate. Morning meditation awakens your spirit, putting you in the best position to deal with aging-related issues throughout the day.

Evening. Take 2 to 5 minutes out of your evening to meditate. Evening meditation helps cleanse your ego of negative thoughts that have built up throughout the day.

Avoid Multitasking

For many people, it gets easier to slow down life and avoid multitasking as they age. Life gets simpler with fewer responsibilities, and a simpler life is a more calming and peaceful life, which allows you to better focus on present moments.

Practice Tai Chi and Qigong

If you are looking for a way to reduce stress and practice mindfulness, consider tai chi or qigong.

Tai chi is an ancient Chinese tradition that is practiced as a graceful form of exercise. It involves a series of movements performed in a slow, focused manner that is combined with deep breathing. Today, tai chi is used for stress reduction and a variety of other health conditions. It is often described as meditation in motion. Tai chi is suitable for older people who may not otherwise exercise, since it is low-impact and does not involve rigorous and intense physical activity. Tai chi requires no special equipment and can be done indoors or outdoors. You can do it alone or in a group class.

Qigong is an ancient Chinese health-care system that integrates physical postures, breathing techniques, and focused attention. It is similar to tai chi. Both qigong and tai chi practices are available in group exercise classes. You can even watch YouTube videos to learn more about the practice. Tai chi and qigong are well suited for people over age 55 because they are low-impact physical activity programs. They also require less stressful stretching than yoga.

Block Out Past Thoughts

Don't compare yourself now to when you were younger and could run a marathon. It is your ego that longs for past accomplishments. Tame your ego to block out past thoughts that are keeping you from living in the present. This was, perhaps, my most difficult challenge. At first, my ego would not accept my cancer diagnosis; I was still living in the past. Yet without acceptance, I could not move forward and effectively battle cancer. Blocking out past thoughts was a difficult but necessary condition for my success.

It's OK to reminisce about your past with a cheerful disposition, but if past memories trigger negative emotions, push your ego off center stage and take control.

Don't Worry about the Future

This is easier said than done, especially if you are battling a life-threatening disease like cancer. Again, tame your ego. If you are frightened by the future—about getting cancer, becoming immobile, losing your hearing, or not being able to eat a big, fat juicy steak—turn these negative emotions into positive emotions. You can do this by blocking out your thoughts about the future and choosing to live only in the present moment.

AN EXCEPTION TO MINDFULNESS

There are exceptions to living in the present. Terminal cancer patients (i.e., stage 4) who are going through trying times in their therapy are prime examples. Their present moment is a horrific one. They need to envision a better future or remember an enjoyable time from the past to feel slightly better. The present moment can be a torment.

When you are at a point of no return and death is near, you may find comfort and peace of mind by reflecting back into the past on parts of your life that were better than what you are experiencing at the present moment.

Final Thoughts

If there was ever a time to live in the present and be free from worries about the past or the future, it is when we are growing old. Living in the present helps us deal with the inconveniences of aging, like life-threatening disease and other severe health conditions, as well as declining physical appearance, bodily functions, and mental health. Achieving mindfulness is certainly one of the keys to practicing positive aging.

CHAPTER FIVE

Positivity

Physical and mental decline are inevitable, but *your* decline is not. Your mind, spirit, and beliefs have a profound influence on the marks of aging and these marks can be reversed by shifts in awareness. I have already shown how the power of mindfulness (living in the present moment) can positively affect your approach toward aging. There is another powerful force to help you age successfully: positivity.

The dictionary defines positivity as the practice of being or tendency to be positive or optimistic in attitude. According to Courtney Ackerman of Positivepsychology.com, "Positive thinking is a mental and emotional attitude that focuses on the bright side of life and expects positive results."[14]

A more pertinent description of positivity in the context of positive aging is given by Kendra Cherry at Verywell Mind (2017): "Positive thinking actually means approaching life's challenges with a positive outlook. It does not necessarily mean avoiding or ignoring the bad things; instead, it involves making the most of the potentially bad situations, trying to see the best in other people and viewing yourself and your abilities in a positive light."[15]

Positivity is different from the Law of Attraction. Positivity is broader and does not depend on the belief in a supernatural force.

The Law of Attraction is the name given to the maxim "like attracts like," which means that focusing on positive or negative thoughts will bring positive or negative experiences into your life. This belief is based upon the idea that people and their thoughts are both made from pure energy, and similar energy vibrations will attract each other.

The Law of Attraction has gained in popularity because of books like *The Secret* and *Ask and It Is Given,* which many people have read as they seek to improve their lives. The relevance here is that people experiencing the inconveniences of aging, including serious disease and the prospects of finality, deal with those issues more successfully with positive thoughts and positive energy.

Law of Attraction believers claim that your thoughts directly influence your health. They believe that worry, fear, stress, or other negative thoughts make people sick, while positive thoughts of wellness or love can keep people healthy and even cure illnesses. They also claim that an important part of maintaining health and curing illness is visualizing yourself being healthy.

Although there are some cases where positive or negative attitudes can produce corresponding results (principally due to the placebo and nocebo effects), there is no scientific basis to the Law of Attraction. In fact, critics have asserted that the evidence provided for substantiating the Law of Attraction is usually anecdotal. Further, the premise that good thoughts attract good things has a flip side: If you have an accident or disease, it's your fault.

I don't know if the Law of Attraction works or not, but I do know positive thoughts are effective tools for successful aging, whether or not there is some supernatural force at work. If the Law of Attraction works for you, look at it as a bonus. In any case, only good comes from a positive attitude.

Practicing positivity matters. If you believe in the power of the Law of Attraction, go with it. If you don't believe in the Law of Attraction, then positivity will still help because it awakens the spirit and pushes the ego off center stage.

Practice Positivity

It's important to recognize how negativity can keep older people from truly living life. I read recently that we have 50,000 to 70,000 unconscious thoughts per day, of which about 80 percent are negative. [16] This certainly makes it seem as if practicing positivity is an uphill climb.

Yet, as we'll discuss, applying positivity to the challenges of aging is quite straightforward—and you can truly transform your life by staying positive. You need to feel good about yourself, no matter what your calendar age is or what mark of aging is challenging you.

According to most research studies, older adults with more positive self-perceptions and views of aging have better physical health and better survival rates than those with more negative self-perceptions and views. Negative views about aging predict low self-esteem and high levels of depression among older adults. (A discussion of positive versus negative self-perceptions is covered in more detail in chapter 15, Aging in America.)

The reason positive thinking is difficult to maintain is that people are impatient and want immediate results. For positivity to be effective, you need to make it a habit. This is accomplished over time by implementing daily positive practices in your life. Here are some habits that you can integrate into your daily life that will help you practice positivity.

Repeat Affirmations

You can use affirmations to establish a healthy habit of positivity. The theory behind some of the affirmations is that the more you say something, the more it imposes itself into your subconscious, where it begins to become reality. In effect, you can reprogram your subconscious mind through daily repetitions of affirmations.

For an older person who is stressed-out about aging, you can repeat an affirmation such as "I feel good about being alive. I feel good about being alive" for a couple of minutes per day. You can repeat this affirmation anytime throughout the day: in the morning, during lunch, or after dinner. You can say your affirmation out loud or silently.

Here is a list of recommended affirmations that are best suited for applying positivity to help better cope with the inconveniences of aging. I used the first four affirmations to help me cope with battling cancer.

Affirmations to Cope with Physical/Mental Decline

I am more than my physical body.
I am great and accept myself as I age.
I feel good about being alive.
I am powerful; I create the life I want.
My spirit strengthens with age.
Life is fun.
I love the challenges that aging presents.
There are no such things as physical problems, only opportunities to
    overcome.
I choose to be happy; I love my life.
I am brave; I am willing to act in spite of aging.
I am OK and accept myself as I age.
I have unlimited power at my disposal.
I am flexible and adapt to change quickly.

Lean on Religious/Supernatural Beliefs

Many people lean on religion or supernatural beliefs to cope with aging and the prospects of finality, and that is OK if it helps you stay positive about your declining life in the physical realm. Belief in the Law of Attraction is a good example of how a supernatural belief can contribute to positivity. With regard to religion, many religious people believe in the power of prayer, which helps them maintain a positive disposition during difficult times.

Again, belief in the supernatural does not have to be proved true (i.e., substantiated by scientific evidence) to help people age successfully. It is the psychological effect of the belief that is important. Having faith in something creates positivity, which helps you deal with the struggles and suffering associated with life and growing old. As long as you don't impose your supernatural beliefs on others, it is likely to yield positive benefits.

Put Yourself in a Happy Place

Imagine that one day a friend convinces you to take a two-day trip to Disney World with other senior citizens. At first you may decline the invitation for fear of the unknown and belief that you won't fit in with the youthfulness of the famous theme park. But you give in to temptation and you are now in the magical kingdom of Disney World. You see children and their parents laughing and eating cotton candy and other delights. You see children screaming happily on roller coasters and other rides, which gives you a personal excitement and rush that you haven't experienced in a long time. You are living vicariously through the adventures of a younger generation of children and adults, or perhaps you even enjoy one of the slower rides at the park yourself. For a moment (or for the entire day), you are carefree and happy to be part of today's youthful world.

We all need to escape from time to time, especially older people who are confined to living quarters. It does not have to be a Disney World trip; it could just be a short trip to the park or the beach or a shopping mall. Placing yourself in a happy place helps generate positive thoughts.

For me, my happy place was taking long walks down a tree-shaded pathway during the early stages of my cancer treatment.

Focus on Something Positive

Focus on things you want to happen in your life. If you pay attention only to the negative things, especially the suffering, stress, and inconveniences associated with the aging process, you are wallowing in your sorrows and not getting any positive nourishment. Positive thoughts are good food for our mind.

Practice avoiding saying or thinking words that are negative, self-defeating, or convey a poor attitude. Instead, replace them with more positive and affirming statements and attitudes.

I focused on the love I had for my wife and children. Every time a negative thought entered my mind, their faces would flood my thoughts and keep me in a positive frame of mind.

Keep a Gratitude Journal

Experiencing gratitude is one of the simplest ways to raise our positive energy. When you recognize that your life is precious, and you acknowledge that aging is a good thing, you will exude positive energy. I've always thought that my 89-year old mother and 96-year-old father have won the biggest lottery of all—an extended life. Now I need to view my life journey in a similar fashion. Appreciating the aging process makes us feel good about ourselves.

I learned the benefits of gratitude rather quickly due to my cancer. You learn to appreciate every day on Earth when you are faced with a life-threatening disease.

Quiet the Ego with Meditation

Meditation quiets the ego, which is naturally biased toward negativity. As we learned in previous chapters, meditation is an effective activity to touch your spirit, which in turn gives off positive vibes. Meditation helps us withdraw attention from stressful, negative patterns we've created over time.

Calm Your Body

Negative emotions get stored in our bodies on a cellular level. Physical motion is one way to release stress and negative energy. It doesn't have to be intense; you can dance, practice yoga or tai chi, or go for a walk.

Final Thoughts

Projecting positivity is easier said than done. It takes effort and consistency to replace negative thoughts with positive thoughts. Practice positivity for a month or two and you will notice changes. You will be more cheerful and happy about your aging life. You will become more confident dealing with the marks of aging. You will be able to take control of the aging process rather than the process controlling you.

To be honest, after my cancer diagnosis, it took me several months before I had positive thoughts. It is difficult to stay positive under trying circumstances, but, if you stick with it, you will succeed.

Suffering (excluding severe pain and terminal disease) is not in the fact itself, but in our perception of the fact. Similarly, aging is a state of mind. You are in control of your attitude every morning you wake up to this lovely world. Maintain positivity by improving the quality of your thoughts, and the quality of your life will improve.

There is a 75-year old study, *The Grant Study of Adult Development*, authored by the Harvard Medical School, that chronicles aging people and happiness.[17] One part of the study specifically follows men aged 55 and older into their 90s, documenting what it is to flourish far beyond conventional retirement. The findings are enlightening for practicing positivity:

- ➤ Our lives continue to evolve in our later years, and often become more fulfilling than before.
- ➤ People who do well in old age did not necessarily do so well in midlife.
- ➤ The credit for growing old with grace and vitality goes more to ourselves than to our genetic makeup.
- ➤ After retirement, stay creative, do new things, learn how to play again.

➢ The way people learn how to cope with life's setbacks makes a difference.

➢ You have to keep your sense of humor, give something of yourself to others, make friends who are younger than you, learn new things, and have fun.

➢ Don't blame others for your problems or deny that you have problems.

➢ A successful old age may lie not so much in our stars and genes as in ourselves.

I know an 85-year old man named Eddie who oozes positivity. Eddie is confined to a wheelchair and has tumors in his stomach and esophagus. He undergoes radiation treatment every week. He is too frail for the tumors to be surgically removed. Eddie tells me that most people he knows try to turn back their odometers (e.g., with antiaging products), but not him. He tells me he is fascinated with his wrinkles—they tell a story of the ups and downs of his life. He also tells me that when he forgets names of people, he laughs about it rather than fretting about it. And on several occasions Eddie opens his bedroom closet door, thinking it's the bathroom, and he laughs some more. Perhaps the most insightful notion Eddie tells me is this: "Being young is awesome, but being old is comfortable."

CHAPTER SIX

The Four A's

I've found that the people who do best with aging are the ones who practice one or more of what I call the Four A's:

➤ Acceptance
➤ Adaptation
➤ Appreciation
➤ Attitude

It has become increasingly evident that our ego and spirit must work together for humans to age successfully. Yes, I've spoken somewhat disparagingly of the ego in earlier chapters, but there is a certain productive role for it to play during the aging process, which I'll describe below. Ego and spirit must come together to practice mindfulness and positivity, and they must coordinate to practice the Four A's.

The Four A's are explained in depth in this chapter, but you will see sidebars with instructions for utilizing one or more of these concepts in subsequent chapters. Look for them under the heading "The A's Have It."

Acceptance

Growing old is a bummer, but you need to accept aging to fully live in your senior years. Once you accept your fate you can better endure the inconveniences of aging and the inevitability of finality. You can enjoy the remainder of your life and appreciate every minute of it. Accepting the notion of growing old sets you up for success.

The people who do the best with aging aren't thinking that much about getting older because they have already accepted their fate. Don't focus on your physical and mental decline; if you do, you are building a scenario where you are not going to age gracefully. Accept the inevitable changes of aging rather than seeing them as abnormal negative events. Inflexible people are miserable and overwhelmed people.

Acceptance is one of the keys to stress-free aging.
Accept your fate.
Accept the need to be pliable.
Accept change.

Adaptation

Remember the first day at a new school when you were a child? Most of us were nervous about entering a new environment, and many of us were apprehensive about the other kids accepting us. Lo and behold, we overcame such obstacles, endured crises, and somehow survived those years—because we adapted.

Adapt to your surroundings as you age, and to your physical and mental handicaps.

If your knees break, use a walker. If your eyes break, wear glasses. If your mind forgets, use a note reminder calendar. If you have cancer, get treatment and hope for the best. It's that simple. This is your encore—make the best of it.

You can learn to adapt to each inconvenience that comes your way. Adapting is one of the keys to improving quality of life as you age.

Be willing to try new things.

Adopt a practical approach to aging.

Put quality of life over shame and embarrassment.

Appreciation

The spirit, and to a lesser extent the ego, can appreciate life as an older person. Gratitude is a necessary component to growing old gracefully. Gratitude means thankfulness, showing your appreciation regarding simple pleasures, and acknowledging everything that you receive. It means living your life as if everything were a miracle and being cognizant of the wonderful things in your life. Gratitude focuses on what is plentiful in your life, rather than what is missing. Research has shown that life improves from the practice of appreciation/gratitude. Giving thanks makes people happier and more resilient, it strengthens relationships, it improves health, and it reduces stress.

Don't get caught up in the daily stresses related to physical and mental decline. Someone once said to me, "Life is rarely perfect, but it's always pretty darn good."

We can learn so much from the elderly rain man who refused my umbrella (in chapter 2, We Are in This Together). I loved his sentiment because he appreciated everything that was good about life. Emulate that man. Appreciate the simple pleasures in life that you previously took for granted. Anyone experiencing a life-threatening disease, as I did with esophageal cancer, knows the true meaning of appreciation. Any cancer survivor will tell you that to live another day is a blessing. That is appreciation at its highest level.

Appreciation improves quality of life. Here are some ways you can practice appreciation:

➤ Imagine completely losing your ability to hear (becoming deaf) and then imagine getting that hearing back. That is what a hearing aid accomplishes—be grateful for hearing aids.
➤ Find pleasure in the small things instead of holding out for big achievements. Be appreciative that you have mobility with a walker rather than desiring the ability to walk again with no assistance.
➤ Put things in their proper perspective. When you are confronted with an inconvenience of aging such as hearing impairment,

rather than dwelling on your inability to hear well, focus your attention on the good that comes from this mark of aging. What you have taken for granted your entire life—sounds— you now have a keen appreciation for that most people do not.

➤ Keep an appreciation journal; write down every day a list of three things for which you are grateful.

➤ Wear an "appreciation" wristband and snap it when you forget to appreciate something in your life.

Attitude

Aging is all about attitude. Attitude is defined as a settled way of thinking or feeling about someone or something and it is typically reflected in a person's behavior. Don't cower to those misguided forever-young attitudes that favor the young over the old. Be proud and honored to have lived this long.

Growing old is not a death sentence—it is a *life* sentence because it pushes us to live. It's about attitude. And if you have a life-threatening disease like cancer, a positive attitude becomes critical for survival. Repeat after me: I will beat cancer.

This is a time when you can put your ego to good use—because having attitude comes naturally to your ego. Have an attitude that older people belong, that older people have value, and that older people are cool. Don't let younger people run all over you; life is too short to put up with that.

I love senior citizens with attitude. At my parents' senior living center, they introduced me to one of their friends, a gentleman named Frank. Frank was sitting in a mobility scooter (a fancy wheelchair) and was wearing a hearing aid.

My mom said, "David, ask Frank how old he is." I thought her request was sort of embarrassing, but I went with it.

"Frank, how old are you?"

Frank replied proudly, "I'm 92 and a half years old."

Frank had a great attitude toward growing old. More of us should proudly display our age.

Aging with a bad attitude is simply out of the question. Here are some suggestions to acquire a positive attitude about aging:

> ➤ Be proud of growing old; it's an achievement that young people admire.
> ➤ Unleash your ego; older people are cool.
> ➤ Remember that growing old is not a death sentence—it's a life sentence.
> ➤ Repeat after me: "I will age with grace."

Final Thoughts

Society perceives senior citizens as over the hill, which suggests they are on the downside of life. But in reality, seniors have lived a life full of experiences, lessons, and learned skills. They have made it to the top of the hill and have earned the right to stay at the top in their golden years. Why go down the hill? It took so long to make it to the top, so stay and enjoy the scenery. This is an attitude shift that benefits every older person.

CHAPTER SEVEN

The Power of Us: Social Support

The power of us comes from both giving and receiving social support. Seniors need to foster both to best engage in positive aging. Social support improves quality of life, and social interaction is a necessary component to your overall well-being.

I've witnessed the extraordinary efforts and compassion of people helping and supporting other people in need—this has made me a true believer in the power of us. Kindness and compassion cost very little for the giver but are priceless to the receiver.

The most striking example of the power of us in recent history is that of the first responders putting their lives in harm's way during the September 11, 2001, attacks on the World Trade Center. Of the 2,977 victims killed in the attacks, 412 were New York City emergency workers who responded to the World Trade Center bombings. This included 343 firefighters, sixty police officers, eight emergency medical technicians and paramedics, and one patrolman from the New York Fire Patrol—they gave their lives saving others.

When I think about Ellen, an 82-year-old widow who lives alone in a modest home in Lynchburg, Virginia, I'm encouraged about the tenderness most people are capable of expressing. Ellen is in declining health, but thanks to a strong support system she won't be alone during her senior years. Her daughter Susie cares for her elderly mother while juggling work and looking after her own three children. Ellen also relies on her church group of women who meet every Tuesday afternoon and participate in social activities like arts and crafts. Living by herself doesn't scare Ellen; she has family and friends to support her.

I'm also heartened by the story of Miss Mary, a lovely 89-year-old lady who was on my Meals on Wheels route in Vero Beach, Florida. Mary lived alone in a tiny house in need of repair. In the three years I delivered hot meals to her, none of her five children visited. Every Tuesday I saw a frail, elderly woman sitting alone in a wheelchair watching overly enthusiastic contestants on *The Price Is Right* on an old tube television. I don't know why her children didn't visit, but she deserved more life than this in her waning years. I suppose some younger people are more concerned with their own lives than with the lives of the people who brought them into this world.

Miss Mary had serious health issues—primarily a heart condition. I knew of two occasions when she required the services of an ambulance. Miss Mary was lonely, so I usually stayed longer just to talk to her. But then something wonderful happened. One Tuesday when I brought her hot meal she was dressed up and lively and happy. I asked her, "What's the occasion?" She told me her grandson was coming to take her to lunch. She smiled at me and said, "Just having someone visit me makes me feel like I exist." Miss Mary broke my heart that day.

The next Tuesday I delivered a meal to Miss Mary, and to my delight her grandson had moved in. He was going to care for her. Miss Mary's quality of life was going to take a big leap forward.

It is interesting how so many animal species intuitively understand the concept of togetherness, while many humans continue to struggle with it. The story of the injured goose illustrates the power of us.

A flock of wild geese had settled to rest on a pond. A farmer had captured one goose and clipped its wings before releasing it. When the flock of geese resumed their flight, the injured goose could not lift itself into the air. The other geese noticed his struggles and flew about in an obvious effort to encourage him, but to no avail.

The entire flock settled back on the pond and waited, even though the urge to continue their journey was strong within them. For several days they waited until the damaged feathers had grown sufficiently to permit the injured goose to fly. Meanwhile, the ashamed farmer watched them as the flock finally rose together and resumed their long flight.

To be fair to us humans, most people, like that flock of geese, care dearly about their family and friends. We just need to work harder at it, so we care about *other* people, particularly those who are aging and injured. We need to integrate caring and responsibility into society and band together as we age. Social support can be a powerful medicine for the elderly and is a necessary component of successful positive aging.

I used to tell a story at business meetings to try to create team unity among my staff. The story is a popular one for team building. Four children are bickering and fighting while their father is dying. They are arguing over who should get his money after he passes. One by one, they give their reasons:

"I should get it, I'm the oldest."

"No, I should get it because I'm the youngest."

"I disagree. I should get it because I'm the strongest."

"No, I should get it because I'm the most hardworking."

The father painfully lifted himself out of bed and left the room in disgust. Minutes later, he came back with four sticks bundled together.

"The child who can break this bundle of sticks gets my money."

Each child tried, but no one could do it, not even the strongest child.

The father took the bundle of sticks and gave each child their individual stick.

"Now, each of you try to break the stick I just gave you."

Each child smiled as they easily snapped their stick in two.

In a scolding voice, the father said, "You are the individual sticks. Alone and unprotected, in times of hardship and trouble, you will snap just like the twig in your hand. But if you learn to get along, support and respect each other, then when you face troubled times and over-whelming obstacles, you will be as strong and powerful as the bunch of sticks that none of you could break."

Social Support Networks Make a Difference

Thankfully, there are many nonprofit organizations in the United States that provide care and compassion for aging adults. These charitable and giving organizations have made significant contributions helping people in need, and they have made a real difference in senior citizens' lives. Here are some examples of organized support groups that matter:

> - Meals on Wheels
> - AARP
> - National Institute on Aging
> - Alliance on Aging Research
> - Alliance for Retired Americans
> - Adult Protection Services
> - Community Care Program
> - Caregiver Action Network
> - Caregiver Support Services
> - Lotsa Helping Hands
> - Alzheimer's Association

These organizations are highly successful in their endeavors. However, on an individual basis, people need their own support networks that matter in their lives. Studies suggest that a personal social network (family and friends) improves quality of life and life expectancy. In the case of a life-threatening condition like cancer, social support (like marriage) matters more than chemotherapy.

Older people who rely on family, friends, and community seem to be happier, doing better, and are better able to get through things. This is the power of us.

Research studies reveal the importance of social networks. More than one in five cancer patients experience loneliness following diagnosis, and those who are lonely are nearly three times more likely to have issues following their treatment plan than those who aren't lonely (31 percent vs. 11 percent).[18]

Among cancer patients who are lonely:

➢ 1 in 30 skipped treatment appointments.
➢ 1 in 17 didn't take medicine as they should.
➢ 1 in 8 were unable to pick up their prescriptions .
➢ 1 in 11 refused some types of treatment.
➢ 1 in 20 refused treatment altogether.

This study strongly suggests that social support is crucial to maintaining quality of life as we age. Social networks matter.

There are attempts to help lonely older adults cope. For example, in 2018 the Kaiser Family Foundation conducted surveys examining the extent of loneliness and social isolation in older adults. Kaiser Permanente is offering pilot programs that will refer lonely or isolated older adults in its region to community services. The effectiveness of this program remains to be seen.[19]

According to testimony to a committee of the National Academies of Sciences by Dr. Linda Fried, Dean of the Mailman School of Public Health, Columbia University, between 33 and 43 percent of older Americans are lonely. And the potential health impacts of loneliness are a higher risk of heart disease, dementia, immune dysfunction, functional impairment, and early death.[20]

Build a Social Support Network

We must try to maintain or build social networks in our senior years. As we age, our circle of friends usually becomes smaller. Some friends die or become incapacitated to the point of not being able to socialize. It is at this point that some of us are in danger of losing our support network. It is important to remain socially engaged. It is particularly difficult to make new relationships after losing a spouse. Avoid living alone in your senior years. Without the support of family and friends, quality of life and life expectancy are compromised.

There are numerous ways to ensure that you will have a social support network as you age:

Family

The most effective way of ensuring social support in your senior years is to maintain close and loving relations with family, particularly your children and siblings. Close family ties help buffer the struggles and the stress of aging in your twilight years.

Friends

Maintaining relations with friends will serve as a powerful support network as you encounter the marks of aging. "You know your real friends in times of a health crisis." I was told this by someone who experienced esophageal cancer before I did. She said, "You will be surprised who your real friends are. The ones who you think are closest may not step up to the plate, while some lesser friends may embrace you in times of need." I found this out during my journey battling cancer. My friends showed their true colors; some disappointed while other exceeded my expectations.

There are a number of ways to meet new friends:

- ➢ Live in a 55+ community
- ➢ Participate in activities such as hiking, dining, and yoga classes.
- ➢ Join a fitness center or a senior center that offers planned activities.
- ➢ Join a bowling league or play golf or tennis.
- ➢ Participate in cards and games groups.
- ➢ Go on group travel trips.

Church and Other Support Organizations

Church is a great place to find support groups for older people, and among the first places you should look. You can also join Internet support groups related to your health concerns (e.g., hearing impairment, dementia). For example, Inspire.com offers access to a variety of online support groups, including online communities for diabetes, digestive system, heart diseases, mental health, behavior, and so on.

Local Organizations/Communities

You can contact local organizations that cater to older people with needs (e.g., Meals on Wheels). Or you can move to a 55+ community or an independent/assisting living facility.

United We Age

Support groups like United We Age offer "Friends for Seniors" services, providing social support to people living alone with no support network (UnitedWeAge.org).

Final Thoughts

There is a popular story about a frail old grandfather who lived with his daughter and son-in-law and their two children. The grandfather's hands trembled, and his vision and hearing were impaired. The family ate dinner together at the table every night. But the old man's shaky hands and failing sight made eating difficult. Meat, potatoes, and vegetables would occasionally fall off his fork onto the floor. His shaky hands made it difficult to grasp larger objects, so he frequently spilled his glass of milk onto the tablecloth.

To minimize the mess, the man's family put all his food in a bowl, but it wasn't sufficient. Over time, the daughter and son-in-law became irritated with spilled milk, noisy eating, and food on the floor. They banished the old man to a small table in the corner of the room to eat alone, while the rest of the family enjoyed dinner.

When the other family members glanced in the grandfather's direction, sometimes he had a tear in his eye as he sat alone. Still, if he spilled his food or drink, his daughter or son-in-law would admonish him. Their two children watched it all in silence.

One evening before supper, the family noticed that the youngest daughter was writing something on two bowls with a magic marker. The father asked his youngest daughter, "What are you making?" The girl replied, "Oh, I am writing 'Mommy' and 'Daddy' on these bowls for you and Mommy to eat your food in when I grow up."

The parents were speechless and then tears started to stream down their cheeks. Though no word was spoken, both knew what must be done.

That evening the husband took the grandfather's hand and gently led him back to the family table. For the remainder of his days, the grandfather ate every meal at the table with the family. Neither husband nor wife seemed to care any longer when a fork was dropped, milk spilled, or the tablecloth soiled.

The power of us starts at home. With every generation, family members grow old, and how they are honored and cared for shapes the attitudes of the next generation of children. Let's show our children how family and friends make a positive difference in an older person's life.

CHAPTER EIGHT

Balance

People who lead well-balanced lives are at peace with themselves, while people who can't seem to find balance lead lives of disarray filled with stress, anxiety, and sometimes depression.

Finding the right balance in your life is important, especially as you grow older and experience the inconveniences of aging. The challenge is that we become increasingly out of balance as we age. We are literally thrown into disequilibrium, which leaves many of us unsettled and confused. Imagine how disruptive hearing impairment or mobility loss is for an older person's lifestyle. Not surprisingly, cancer threw me out of balance—both emotionally and physically.

The tools for positive aging—your spirit, tapping your social network, and practicing mindfulness, positivity, and the Four A's—can help you confront life-threatening diseases, illnesses, and changes in physical appearance, bodily function, and mental health. You need to constantly tweak your life to smooth out the emotional roller coaster of aging. This is what I mean by balance.

Balancing one's life includes simple things as well as complex things. I have learned that when my stomach makes as much noise as my coffeemaker after a hearty meal, it's time to change my diet. This is a simple problem with a simple solution. However, when some of us experience depression because of diminished self-worth due to aging or because we've been diagnosed with a serious illness, the problem and solution of balancing becomes more complex.

As we age and grow more out of balance, many of us are slow to adjust. And for those who do attempt to re-balance, many times our actions are misguided and misplaced. This occurs because the ego orchestrates rebalancing, and it seeks temporary and superficial solutions like traveling to Egypt to visit the pyramids to fulfill a bucket list item.

Achieving life balance is more profound than filling up bucket lists. As older people, we need to better understand our physical and mental strengths and weaknesses, so we can place greater emphasis on our strengths and repair our weaknesses. Many of us enter our senior years with the same set of values, priorities, and expectations that we possessed as younger adults. We need to re-balance the composition of our life "portfolio" to better fit the new reality of being an older person. (For more on this, see the Life Balancing Audit presented in Chapter 14, A Lifestyle Plan for Positive Aging.)

The challenge with balancing is not so much in talking about it, but in achieving it and maintaining it over time. As we age and emotional problems arise, it is often a sign that an imbalance is present. Without proper balancing, aging will get the best of us.

Ways to Re-balance

There are five major categories for rebalancing as you age:

> ➤ Expectations
> ➤ Coping skills
> ➤ Lifestyle
> ➤ Social interactions
> ➤ Priorities

Most people tend to focus on one aspect more than the others. For example, you may find that your focus is on your lifestyle (e.g., healthy diet and exercise), while paying little attention to your social interaction with family and friends. There is no optimal balance; it is up to each individual to find his or her balance among life's categories. Here are some ways to re-balance your life as you age.

Expectations

Confronting your expectations as you age is perhaps the most important balancing act of your life. Experiencing physical and mental decline triggers endless rounds of revising expectations about your changing physical and mental realities, making this a balancing act of great proportions.

The practice of positive aging requires that we possess positive beliefs and expectations regarding aging. According to a recent study conducted by Aili Breda and Amber Watts, there is a positive correlation between positive beliefs/expectations and favorable physical/mental health and longevity.[21]

But managing expectations is nontrivial from an older person's perspective. I believe there are times when having low or zero expectations rather than positive expectations is the more attractive route for confronting many of the inconveniences of aging that life throws at us. I label these expectations "rational expectations." In economics, rational expectations theory states that when making decisions, individuals will base their decisions on the best information available and learn from past trends. Rational expectations are the best guess for the future.

We need to make use of all the available information, as well as past trends about our physical and mental decline as we age. So, if we have serious arthritis, we need to lower our expectations of the type of physical activities we can do. But if we have Parkinson's disease—based on the available information on Parkinson's disease and based on past trends of our physical decline due to Parkinson's disease—the rational decision may be to eliminate expectations completely and create a decision matrix of possibilities.

Any expectation for a person living with Parkinson's disease may result in disappointment and frustration. But believing in possibilities eliminates preconceived notions of what might happen in the future. It's like hedging your bets; choosing from a long list of possibilities lowers the likelihood of failure (disappointment). This is especially applicable for individuals facing serious physical or mental decline.

Of course, high expectations when we are young adults filled with hopes and desires makes sense because high expectations give us a goal to aim at to achieve our goals in life. But from a happiness perspective—for even young adults—high expectations may set you up for inevitable disappointment. That is the assertion Barry Schwartz makes in his book *The Paradox of Choice*.[22] His assertion is that "everything was better back when everything was worse. His reasoning is that when everything was worse, it was possible for people to have experiences that were a pleasant surprise. If we have high expectations, the best you can ever hope for is that stuff is as good as you expect it to be. You will never be pleasantly surprised, because your expectations are too high. The secret to happiness is low expectations. He goes on to state that wanting to do more is commendable, and achieving lofty goals is personally exciting, but if you can settle for staying healthy and calm—that is happiness. From a mental health perspective, if you do not have high expectations, then you will not be disappointed when they are not achieved because they never existed. This creates a more stress-free mode of behavior for individuals, especially for older persons.

The positive correlation between rational expectations and happiness applies nicely to the plight of older persons. The objective while aging is not to change and manage expectations, but to free yourself from having expectations—or keep them at low, rational levels.

People need to confront aging without the pressure of living up to preconceived notions. When things don't materialize the way you expected, you need to realize this is how life works rather than becoming frustrated at the outcome. Confront aging with an open mind and you will minimize disappointment and heartache.

You need to let go of any anguish, shame, or insecurity you might feel because of failed expectations over aging. According to Buddhist thought, expectations are almost always the result of a "wanting mind" that is driven by desire, aversion, and anxiety. The path toward freeing yourself from these wants and expectations is to know what is true in the present moment. You make decisions based on the best information available to you, as well as past trends.

Expectations are future-based and assume a certain result. Expectations hold your present sense of self-worth hostage to a future that may or may not happen. From a rational expectation perspective, the solution is to lower your expectations considerably or, more on point, replace expectations with *possibilities*. Possibilities reflect your preferences for the future, realizing that the future is unknown and open to an infinite number of prospects. Since you have no pre-conceived notions (expectations) of what will occur in the future, you are better able to respond to events affecting your life.

For example, if you are happy playing tennis three times per week with other senior tennis players, and you fall and break your hip, which ends your days as a tennis player—how will you respond? If you are free of expectations and focus on possibilities, you will be able to do exactly what life calls for in the moment. You would be able to let go of your goal of playing tennis and move on with a positive attitude about life without tennis. The disappointment of never playing tennis again is kept to a minimum. And your list of possibilities might include golf and card games.

Employ rational expectations about how you think aging affects your life and you will have a more balanced life filled with adventure and possibilities.

Coping Skills

Coping skills are essential for navigating the struggles and occasional suffering associated with aging. These skills are indispensable elements in maintaining balance in our lives. Just as teenagers need to learn coping skills for dealing with the ups and downs of life, older people need coping skills to deal with the challenging aspects of aging.

A COPING LESSON

I'm reminded of a story my sister told me about her 19-year old son. He was the proud owner of a used BMW automobile. One day, he got a flat tire and realized that his BMW was not equipped with a spare tire. What he didn't know was that BMWs are equipped with run-flat tires that are designed to resist the effects of deflation when punctured. He called his mom in a panic and screamed, "I don't know what to do!" His mom calmly told him to take his car to an automobile repair shop. Her son replied in a high-pitched voice, "They don't know how to work on BMWs!"

His mom calmly told him not to worry, just take the car to a BMW repair shop.

Son: "I don't know where there are any BMW shops. I can't handle this! You need to drive here and help me!"

Mom: "No, I'm not driving to you. You need to take care of this yourself. Just Google "BMW" in your location and it will identify BMW repair shops."

Son: "No, I can't do that—there are no BMW repair shops around here. I'm just going to leave my car here. I need to go home."

In the end, he took his car to the nearest gas station, only to find out that his car was equipped with run-flat tires. The next day he purchased a new tire at his BMW dealership. Suffice it to say, my sister's son had little to no coping skills at the time. He was not equipped to meet the challenges of a flat tire. The good news is that he learned from his flat tire experience and is more prepared to cope with not only future automobile problems, but with the obstacles life hands us as we age.

To cope with problems in your life, you need to be able to:

➤ Manage stress.
➤ Exhibit positivity under trying circumstances.
➤ Exhibit patience.
➤ Find humor in the situation.

Coping skills help maintain your mental and emotional health under the best and worst situations. Here are some ways to develop coping skills:
➤ Stay positive while minimizing negative thoughts when confronted with a challenge.
➤ Stay calm.
➤ Seek support from others.
➤ Don't overwork; be efficient in utilizing your energy on a particular problem.

People with poor coping skills lead stressful lives, and this especially applies to older people facing the challenges of aging.

According to Dr. Hans-Werner Wahl and Dr. Laura Gitlin's presentation "Aging: Changing Attitudes and Successful Coping Mechanisms," "Incorporating coping skills into your everyday life helps reduce functional disabilities and enhance self-efficacy. As a result, increased well-being and health can lead to higher life expectancy."

Learning new coping skills as we age is necessary and challenging because the deterioration to our physical functions is new to us. We have no prior experience in how to deal with such conditions as hearing or mobility loss or a heart condition. How we individually cope with physical and mental decline affects our quality of life as we grow old. Acquiring the right coping skills is critical to living a more balanced and joyous life in our senior years.

Lifestyle

The inconveniences of aging require that you make lifestyle changes to maintain balance in your life. So many people continue with lifestyles that they've grown accustomed to and enjoyed as younger people with younger bodies. Sometimes it is difficult to break a habit.

Monitor your lifestyle and make adjustments that better align with your aging life. Positive lifestyle choices create a healthier disposition and boost self-confidence as you deal with the inconveniences of aging. Here are some of the elements of lifestyle you need to monitor and change as you confront your own inconveniences of aging.

Maintain a healthy diet. As people age, their digestive systems age as well, which triggers a host of digestive health issues such as heartburn, constipation, diarrhea and frequent urination. Follow a healthy dietary regimen to minimize digestive disruptions. So many people stubbornly eat foods that cause digestive problems.

MY JOURNEY

My post-surgery body has resulted in significant lifestyle changes. In fact, my eating and sleeping habits have been turned upside down and inside out. Due to my post-surgery stomach complications, I am mostly on a diet of liquids and soft foods (e.g., fish). I am now forced to sleep on a 45-degree incline because my rearranged stomach no longer has a flap valve to keep its contents (e.g., bile and acid) from overflowing into my esophagus and mouth. For a year after my surgery, I was hooked up to a feeding tube due to complications with my stomach's ability to move food to my intestines.

Healthy choices. The inconveniences of aging require older adults to make some practical choices about daily living. For example, sleep problems are a common inconvenience among older people, so you may have to change your sleep regimen (e.g., avoiding eating heavy meals and limiting your intake of alcohol, caffeine, and nicotine before bedtime). Perhaps you need to make practical adjustments to your life due to hearing impairment. Since it is difficult to hear conversations in a noisy, crowded room such as a diner, you may choose to socialize in quieter restaurants and avoid attending crowded social gatherings.

Regularly exercise. The benefits of regular exercise are plentiful for older people, including reducing stress, improving memory retention, and promoting more restful sleep. Of course, the exercise routines for an older person are quite different from those for a younger person. Rather than run for 30 minutes on a treadmill, which is hard on the knees, you may consider walking on a treadmill for 45 minutes, which is much easier on the knees and other joints. Switching to less-impact exercises like walking, swimming, and balance exercises is a wise decision as we age.

However, exercise guru Dean Rosson strongly recommends that older people engage in weight-resistance exercises. He recommends working out with light weights 3 to 5 times per week.[23]

Activities. Staying active is a requirement for maintaining long-term health, and it is an effective tool for balancing your life. You may have to play less tennis if your knees ache. Some people replace tennis with golf or pickleball since they are less physically stressful activities. A routine of playing card games or arts and crafts is preferable to a sedentary routine of watching television.

Fashion/Attire. As we age, our bodies become more sensitive to temperature changes. For many older people, our bones and joints ache, which makes walking a chore. Wearing sweaters to protect against the cold of air-conditioned buildings, soft shoes such as sneakers (ladies, throw away those stilettos!), looser clothing for comfort, and hats for sun protection are practical fashion statements for older people.

Organization. I've found that organized people live less stressful lives than people who are disorganized—and this is especially true for people with memory loss. Following daily routines and doing less multitasking creates a simpler way of life that is what many of us strive for as we age.

Rest. When I was a younger man, I was embarrassed to take naps in the middle of the day. And so many of us continue to resist rest as we begin to age. We need to change this mindset. People are biologically programmed to sleep not only for a long period in the middle of the night but also for a short period in the middle of the day. So, if you don't feel fully alert during the day, a nap may be just what you need. For many older people, taking a brief nap can provide the needed energy to perform fully for the rest of the day.

Social Interactions

Social life changes dramatically as you age. Your circle of friends usually becomes smaller. This is especially evident when we enter our 70s, 80s, and 90s—friends die, or become incapacitated to the point of not being able to socialize.

As you age, it is important to remain socially involved to maintain your mental health. Humans are social beings and most people feel better when interacting with others. Socializing helps keep your mind sharp and even prevents depression and postpones dementia. Many studies point to the importance of frequent social participation for maintaining quality of life.

For many of us, our social lives get more out of balance with each passing year. It is particularly difficult for those elderly people who have been unsociable most of their lives to begin to engage in social activities. Similarly, it may be difficult to make new relationships after losing a spouse. Some of us live lonely lives in our senior years, but it doesn't have to be this way. With the right adjustments, older adults can successfully transition to a social life more aligned with senior living.

Social balancing varies, depending on your stage in senior life. A 67-year-old person has different social needs from an 85-year-old person living in a senior living facility. The objective is to adjust your social life to minimize the emotional ups and downs of aging for your life situation.

There are many ways you can interact socially throughout your senior years.

Participate in group activities. Look online for aging boomer's groups for hiking and dining, or even meditation and yoga classes. Contact your local fitness center, town hall, or information center for ideas of groups that meet in your community. Senior centers exist to help ease the transition of aging by planning activities such as exercise, meals, games, and trips.

Attend church or other support organizations. Church is a great place to find support groups for older people.

Spend time with family and friends. Place greater emphasis on your relationships with family and friends. When we were younger, many of us were more concerned about how people perceived us than how we generally felt about ourselves. We cared about how we appeared socially, climbing social ladders, befriending important people, driving cars that impressed others, and so forth. As we age, this kind of attitude creates an imbalance that needs correction. We need to become more focused on the authenticity of our relationships than with social status.

Love yourself. Spend more time with yourself and less time with superficial relationships. Loving yourself as you age raises self-worth, which touches your spiritual side.

Get out more. As we age, some of us tend to socialize less. Some alone time is healthy, but an excessive amount is unhealthy. Become aware of your activities with people, animals, and nature and maintain a reasonable level of social interaction.

Priorities

We all prioritize our time whether we know it or not, but identifying the right priorities is not as easy as it may sound. As young adults, work and raising a family were our top priorities. But as we age, retire and become empty nesters, a job and raising a family are erased from our priority list, which leaves many of us feeling empty and unsettled. Reprioritizing your life is essential for successful aging. If your priorities are not aligned correctly with your new life experiences, chances are you will end up feeling unsatisfied and disappointed with your life.

So, how do you reprioritize your life?

It is important to have a vision for how you want to spend the rest of your life so you can identify which activities to de-emphasize and which activities move you toward your vision. A vision keeps you grounded about your priorities. Your vision may be focused on fulfilling some things you want to achieve in your senior years. For example, it may be important to you to travel more while you are physically able. Or you may want to spend more time with community service rather than playing cards with friends. Experiencing cancer certainly changed my priorities in life. I value health and relationships a great deal more today than I did before cancer.

Next, make a list of everything that is important to you that aligns with your vision. This list can include items like family and friends, religion, relationships, activities, diet and exercise, alone-time (rest), community service, and work. Sort these items into the following four priority categories.

➢ Well-being
➢ Social Interaction
➢ Goals
➢ Happiness

Put your list in order based on how important each item is to you. This becomes your priority list.

What do you spend most of your time doing? If it's not a top priority item, then why are you spending your time on it? Identifying how you spend your time helps you reprioritize your changing life. You will be able to better allocate your time and energy to the things that matter and avoid spending time on things that no longer matter.

Final Thoughts

As we grow older and experience many of the inconveniences of aging, it is helpful to conduct a personal audit of yourself to see if you feel balanced. Aging leaves many of us feeling unsettled, anxious, and confused about who we are and what our purpose is. It is not surprising that so many older people get more and more out of balance with their lives.

Balanced living is when you can always offset any negative events in your life with positive ones. Simplicity is also an important part of balancing your life, especially for older people. People who are successful at aging simplify their lives and reduce the number of out-of-balance things that can disrupt joyful living.

A balanced life takes you closer to a spiritual life, so it becomes easier to cope with the inconveniences of aging. You can be at peace with yourself and love the person you are at this late stage in life. If you put the time and effort into rebalancing your life as you age, your twilight years will truly be happy and contented.

CHAPTER NINE

The Inconveniences of Aging

In the end, life is about how you deal with the hand you are dealt. If you live long enough, you will, due to physical and mental decline, encounter a long and varied list of "inconveniences"—life-threatening diseases and illnesses, hearing impairment, loss of sex drive, mobility problems, etc. How you prepare for and battle against each inconvenience is what determines the quality of your life, both physically and emotionally.

If you are diagnosed with cancer, heart disease, Parkinson's disease, or Alzheimer's disease, are you emotionally prepared to battle and endure? If your knees fail, are you emotionally prepared to use a walker? Do you have the confidence to wear a hearing aid in public? Are you too vain to handle the onset of wrinkles and age spots on your face? Are you mentally prepared to say good-bye to your youthful appearance forever?

A List Too Long

Aging does not discriminate. All people experience physical and mental decline: rich and poor; male and female; white and black and all the colors in between—it makes no difference.

Below are the inconveniences of aging, and I expect most people to relate to some, or even many of these marks of aging. It's a long list, but it's not an exhaustive list by any means. Please add to it if you'd like. I've divided the list into four categories: diseases and illnesses; bodily functions; mental health; and physical appearance.

Following these four lists, I provide a deeper examination of seven of these inconveniences, how they affect the quality of our lives, and some ways to address the maladies or their symptoms by presenting current treatments and recommended coping methods practicing positive aging. These inconveniences reflect the four major categories of the marks of aging: disease, bodily functions, mental health, and physical appearance.

THE A'S HAVE IT

Acceptance. You must accept your fate in life and be willing to pass the baton to younger people. It is their turn. It is OK because you are now on another journey filled with peace and contentment. Further, if you truly believe you are more than your physical body, it is easier to accept the physical and mental changes that inevitably occur as you age.

Diseases and Illnesses

Many of us eventually experience true suffering in the form of diseases and illnesses. These are the most difficult of the inconveniences of aging—they are the true suffering of aging. Here are just a handful of them:

Heart disease. Heart disease is the number one cause of death among adults over the age of 60. Heart disease includes conditions such as heart failure, heart attack, and heart arrhythmia, which can cause the heart to beat ineffectively and impair circulation. Heart disease is associated with or caused by, diabetes, high blood pressure, smoking, improper diet, and lack of exercise. It can also have a genetic component.

Cancer. Cancer can come in many forms, including breast cancer, colon cancer, and skin cancer, as well as malignant blood and bone marrow diseases that cause leukemia. It is the second-leading cause of death among seniors. Many cancers occur at a higher rate among older adults, though the cause for that is not clear. Cancers can also be more difficult to treat due to other health conditions that may also be present.

Chronic obstructive lung disease (COPD). Chronic obstructive lung disease decreases the lungs' ability to exchange carbon dioxide for oxygen. As the disease progresses, patients have to work harder and harder to breathe and often may feel as if they are suffocating. This disease is often linked to a lifetime of smoking, but it can be due to environmental factors.

Pneumonia. Pneumonia is the fifth-highest killer of older adults and is especially deadly during the winter months of flu season. Seniors with chronic diseases such as diabetes, heart disease, and respiratory conditions are at higher risk for developing pneumonia. Flu and pneumonia shots are recommended for all adults over the age of 55 to help prevent this killer.

Parkinson's disease. Parkinson's disease is a chronic neurological disorder that affects nerve cells in the part of the brain that controls muscle movement.

Diabetes. Having high blood glucose levels is the hallmark of diabetes, a group of diseases that affects the body's ability to produce or use insulin correctly.

Osteoporosis. Osteoporosis is a condition that causes bones to break more easily and take longer to heal. As a result, even minor falls can land seniors in the hospital.

Coronavirus (COVID-19). At the time of this writing in the spring of 2020, the coronavirus is a true pandemic, having spread to virtually every nation in the world. COVID-19 seems to have a higher mortality rate than common illnesses such as the seasonal flu. Severe complications or even death are more common with the elderly as well as with people suffering from a suppressed immune system or an underlying heart or lung disease.

Bodily Functions

Digestive health. More than 40 percent of older people experience one or more digestive problems every year.

Urination. People may urinate more as they get older due to medical problems like prostate enlargement in men and continence problems in women.

Arthritis. The probability of a senior citizen getting a chronic illness such as arthritis is as high as getting a common cold.

Mobility. The loss of mobility might be the most humbling of inconveniences.

Falling. Falls are the leading cause of injury and death for old people. Please, do not fall!

Pain. The one thing nearly all older people have in common is pain (e.g., back and neck pain, bone spurs, frozen shoulder).

Hearing. By age 75, 48 percent of men and 37 percent of women experience hearing impairment. However, only one in five of them wear a hearing aid. Further, many older people experience tinnitus, which is the perception of a noise or ringing in the ears. Tinnitus affects about 15 to 30 percent of people.

Vision. As you age beyond 50 you may notice the need for more frequent changes in your eyeglass prescription. Lenses get thicker and thicker, but there is an end in sight.

Smelling. Are you no longer able to smell odors well? A person's sense of smell gets muted with age.

Tasting. A person's sense of taste diminishes rapidly around age 80.

Voice. Vocal cords change as the larynx ages, which alters the sounds of older people's voices.

Sleeping. According to some surveys, 88 percent of people over 74 reported sleep complaints.

Stamina. With age, we lose muscle tissue and our muscles become more rigid, resulting in reduced stamina.

Sex drive. Sex drive decreases as you age, especially for men and women over 60, but it doesn't have to end.

Mental Health

Memory loss. Memory loss surfaces in people over 50 and can lead to more serious mental health issues.

Dementia. Have you ever experienced that awkward moment when someone asks you to tell them about yourself and you are speechless? Dementia is a general loss in intellectual abilities serious enough to interfere with daily life. Alzheimer's disease is the most common form of dementia.

Depression. Depression is far too common among older people. About 6.5 million senior citizens have been diagnosed as depressed. (See chapter 1, Why Positive Aging?)

Anxiety. Anxiety disorders are common as people grow older. Acute anxiety can be disruptive to your life, but it is treatable.

Physical Appearance

Changes in physical appearance may sound like superficial inconveniences of aging, but they create a great deal of concern and anxiety among people experiencing them.

Turkey neck. A turkey neck is what happens when the skin underneath your chin becomes loose and lax, resembling a turkey's wattle.

Turkey arms. Turkey arms are the turkey neck's cousin. The skin of your underarms becomes loose and lax. Saggy arm flesh is especially a problem for older women.

Wrinkles. Is your skin losing elasticity, becoming drier, more lined, and wrinkled?

Age spots, skin tags, blemishes. It doesn't seem to end.

Shrinkage. You are not imagining it; you are shrinking.

Bones/joints. Old bones not only talk, they thin and shrink.

Drooping nose/ears. Ears and nose sag and droop with age, which causes them to lengthen.

Unusual hair growth. Hair sprouts in the most unwanted places: ears, nose, and face.

Hair loss. Bald is beautiful and thinning is winning.

Graying. Distinguished or old, there are 50 shades of it.

Excessive weight gain/loss. Are you aging in a big way? Like adding 20 to 80 pounds? Or are you losing a lot of weight and becoming frail? Both excessive weight gain and weight loss are common as we age.

Dental. A variety of serious dental health issues arise as we age.

A Closer Look

Let's take a closer look at seven of the inconveniences listed above: cancer, dementia, depression, declining mobility, hearing impairment, wrinkles, and coronavirus. Although I present ideas about treatment/ remedies for each inconvenience, ultimately, these marks are likely to become permanent struggles or source of suffering for many as they age.

It may not be possible to cure or eliminate these maladies. Therefore, it is important to learn to live with them by tapping into the ideas and techniques presented in the previous chapters, such as inner spirit, mindfulness, positivity, the Four A's, social support, and balance.

Please note that the treatments and remedies presented for each inconvenience are those recommended by medical professionals in sources like WebMD, the National Institute of Health, the Mayo Clinic.

Cancer

Let's begin with what so far has been my greatest inconvenience of aging: cancer.

Cancer is a genetic disease caused by changes to genes that control the way our cells function, especially how they grow and divide. In all types of cancer, some of the body's cells begin to divide without stopping and spread into surrounding tissues. As cells become more and more abnormal, old or damaged cells survive when they should die, and new cells form when they are not needed. These extra cells can divide without stopping and may form growths called tumors.

Cancerous tumors are malignant, which means they can spread into, or invade, nearby tissues. In addition, as these tumors grow, some cancer cells can break off and travel to distant places in the body through the blood or the lymph system and form new tumors far from the original tumor.

A cancer that has spread from the place where it first started to another place in the body is called metastatic cancer. The process by which cancer cells spread to other parts of the body is called metastasis.

Types of Cancer

There are more than 100 types of cancer. Specific types of cancer are usually named for the organs or tissues where the cancers initially form. For example, lung cancer starts in cells of the lung and brain cancer starts in cells of the brain. My esophageal cancer started in cells in my esophagus. Some cancers may be described by the type of cell that formed them, such as an epithelial cell or a squamous cell. Specific types of cells where cancer originates are: carcinoma, sarcoma, leukemia, lymphoma, multiple myeloma, and melanoma.

Stages of Cancer

Stage refers to the extent of your cancer, such as how large the tumor is, and if it has spread.

Stage 0: Abnormal cells are present but have not spread to nearby tissue.

Stages 1, 2, 3: Cancer is present. The higher the number, the larger the cancer tumor and the likelihood it has spread into nearby tissues.

Stage 4: The cancer has spread to distant parts of the body.

Impact of Cancer

Below is a list of the cancer types that were diagnosed with the greatest frequency (40,000 cases per year or more) in the United States in 2018, excluding nonmelanoma skin cancers. Cancer incidence and mortality statistics are also presented.[24]

Estimated numbers of new cases and deaths for each common cancer type:

Cancer Type	Estimated New Cases	Estimated Deaths
Bladder	80,470	17,670
Breast (Female – Male)	268,600 – 2,670	41,760 – 500
Colon and Rectal (Combined)	145,600	51,020
Endometrial	61,880	12,160
Kidney (Renal Cell and Renal Pelvis) Cancer	73,820	14,770
Leukemia (All Types)	61,780	22,840
Lung (Including Bronchus)	228,150	142,670
Melanoma	96,480	7,230
Non-Hodgkin Lymphoma	74,200	19,970
Pancreatic	56,770	45,750
Prostate	174,650	31,620
Thyroid	52,070	2,170

Treatment Options

The primary treatment options for cancer are:

- Surgery
- Chemotherapy
- Radiation therapy
- Immunotherapy

Other procedures include targeted therapy, stem cell transplants, hyperthermia, photodynamic therapy, blood product donation and transfusion, and lasers.

Surgery

Many people with cancer are treated with surgery. Surgery may be open or minimally invasive. Surgery works best for solid tumors that are contained in one area. It is usually a local treatment, which means that it treats only the part of your body with the cancer.

Radiation Therapy

Radiation therapy (also called radiotherapy) is a cancer treatment that uses high doses of radiation to kill cancer cells and shrink tumors.

Chemotherapy

Chemotherapy is a type of cancer treatment that uses drugs to kill cancer cells. Chemotherapy works by stopping or slowing the growth of cancer cells, which grow and divide quickly. A wide variety of chemotherapy treatments have been developed to treat the many types of cancer. Most often, you will have chemotherapy along with other cancer treatments.

Immunotherapy

Your immune system, which helps your body fight infections and other diseases, is made up of white blood cells and the organs and tissues of the lymph system. Immunotherapy is a type of biological therapy that uses substances made from living organisms to help your immune system fight cancer.

Immunotherapy is not yet as widely used as surgery, chemotherapy, and radiation therapy. However, a variety of immunotherapies have been approved to treat people with many types of cancer. Many other immunotherapies are being studied in clinical trials, which are research studies involving people. Different forms of immunotherapy may be given in different ways, including intravenous, oral, topical, and intravesical.

COPING WITH CANCER

The coping skills presented in the previous chapters are essential in dealing with a disease as serious as cancer. Based on my experience with esophageal cancer, I will share some of the complications and troublesome side effects stemming from my cancer and how I coped with them.

Shame and embarrassment. When I was first diagnosed with cancer, my initial emotional response was of shame and embarrassment. Cancer brands you; public perception places a stigma on people struck with the disease. Cancer was a hit to my ego—I was embarrassed to tell friends that I had cancer. In time, I learned to tap into my spirit and tame my ego. As I strengthened my spirit via activities like meditation, walking, and writing (this book), shame and embarrassment withered away.

Anxiety and depression. I experienced both anxiety and depression during my chemotherapy/radiation treatment and for several months post-surgery. Aside from medications, there are other ways to lessen the effects of depression and anxiety. Practicing mindfulness and positivity lessened the magnitude of my depression and anxiety about cancer. And today, living in the present moment lessens my anxiety about the future (worrying about my future health). Repeating affirmations about the good things in my life helps me control my depressive thoughts.

Physical decline. I experienced thinning hair, gagging and vomiting, and weight loss (30 pounds) due to my battle with cancer. Dramatic changes to my body were difficult to handle. Losing 25 pounds and approaching an emaciated state seriously lowered my self-image and self-esteem. I refused to go out in public and be seen.

Coping with physical decline is not trivial, but I learned to cope by embracing acceptance. Accepting the notion that cancer changed my life forever sets me up for success. Since my stomach is now half its original size, I will be a thinner man compared to my former self. Acceptance is the key to my survival and future happiness.

Facing prospects of death. Cancer introduced the fear of dying into my everyday life. Before my diagnosis, I shied away from the prospects of my finality. Don't we all? But battling cancer changed me; I now recognize that death is close. Coping with awareness of my own mortality is not easy. Most people lean on religion or adopt supernatural beliefs about the afterlife. I lean more heavily on the belief that I am more than my physical body. I find comfort in the belief that my spirit lives on after death. However, I have realized that perhaps the best way to cope with mortality is to accept and appreciate the moments we have in life. Do not live in fear of death; instead embrace every moment as if it were your last.

Balance. Cancer threw me off my game; I got out of balance both emotionally and physically. Without proper balance, stress, anxiety, and depression filled my life. Changes in lifestyle and expectations have been necessary conditions for my survival and to sustain a good quality of life.

As I mentioned previously, my lifestyle is quite different today. I live on a liquid and soft food diet. I sleep on a 45 degree incline to keep the bile from flowing out of my stomach. I no longer socialize as much as before my cancer diagnosis due to some insecurities still present in me.

My only hope for living a balanced life is to revise my expectations of what life is. I am no longer a young, healthy male with a long future ahead of me. Confronting our expectations as we age or face serious disease is perhaps the most important balancing act of our life. Expectations for a person like me with a physical handicap and the possibility of a cancer encore could set me up for inevitable disappointment. Do I really want to have expectations of a normal life after esophageal cancer treatment and surgery? I would likely be disappointed and disillusioned. I must free myself of expectations. I remind myself that expectations are not in the present; they are future-based and assume a certain result.

> My solution is to replace expectations with *possibilities*. Possibilities are based in the present moment. In my present condition, I realize that my future is unknown. I don't know what I'll be able to do or how long I will do it.
>
> Free of expectations, I respond to what life has handed me in the present moment. The pleasant result? I now have a life filled with new adventures and possibilities.

Final Thoughts

Cancer is personal to me—will battle it for the rest of my life. Even though I'm cancer-free due to chemotherapy, radiation, and surgery, cancer can always come back. However, as long as I'm on this Earth enjoying life with a support network of family and friends, cancer and my other physical complications, including the usual marks of aging, are merely inconveniences.

Dementia

Cognition is the reasoning, awareness, perception, knowledge, intuition, and judgment that we possess. These are skills we need to think, talk, learn, and read. Dementia affects cognition.

Dementia is a general term for memory loss and the diminishment of other intellectual abilities that are serious enough to interfere with daily life. Dementia can be caused by various disorders that affect parts of the brain involved with thought processes. Its prevalence increases in old age from about 10 percent at age 65 to about 50 percent over age 85. Alzheimer's disease, specifically, is the most common cause of dementia, accounting for about 50 percent of cases. Other forms of dementia include vascular dementia and dementia with Lewy bodies.

Dementia is *not* a normal part of aging. It is different from the age-related memory loss that is common in older people. Dementia is said to be early onset if it comes on before the age of 65.

Demented behavior can include wandering, physical aggression, verbal outbursts, depression, and psychosis. Other symptoms include memory problems, language problems, disorientation, changes in mood/behavior, and problems during daily activities. Symptoms tend to develop slowly, often over several years. In the early stages of the disease, many people are able to cope. As the disease progresses, care and outside support are usually needed.

In the later stages of dementia, speech may be lost and severe physical problems may develop, including problems with mobility, incontinence, and general frailty. Some people can live for many years after dementia has been diagnosed.

Types of Dementia

Alzheimer's disease is the most common form of dementia. It affects over 5 million people and causes about half of all dementia cases. Over time, people with Alzheimer's disease have trouble thinking clearly. They find it hard to do everyday things like shopping, driving, and cooking. As the illness progresses, people with Alzheimer's disease may need someone to take care of all their needs at home or in a nursing home. These needs may include feeding, bathing, and dressing.

Vascular dementia is a medical condition that causes serious memory problems. Memory loss and confusion are caused by small strokes or changes in the blood supply to the brain. Vascular dementia causes about a quarter of all cases of dementia.

Dementia with Lewy bodies is the second most common type of progressive dementia. It causes a progressive decline in mental abilities. It may also cause visual hallucinations and can result in unusual behavior such as having conversations with deceased loved ones. In this type of dementia, protein deposits, called Lewy bodies, develop in nerve cells in regions of the brain involved in thinking, memory, and movement (motor control).

Treatment for Dementia

According to one dementia study, there are nine risk factors for developing dementia[25]: lack of education, hypertension, obesity, hearing loss, smoking, depression, physical inactivity, diabetes and social isolation. The study's authors argue that, in general, medications have proved ineffective at curing or stopping the disease and its most common form, Alzheimer's disease. But the good news is that we have more control over our cognitive health than we previously believed. The study asserts that if we live a healthier lifestyle based on the nine risk factors they identified, we may be able to lower the risk of developing dementia in our lives.

Here are some of the ways to lower the risk of contracting dementia:

Exercise. Aerobic exercise of at least 30 minutes is good for brain health.

Eat foods for a healthy brain. Although there are no conclusive studies on the correlation between food and brain health, here are some of the foods that people associate with brain health: beans, green peas, grain products, cereal, oranges, limes, lemons, sweet peppers, strawberries, cantaloupes, tomatoes, broccoli, leafy greens, almonds, avocado, fish, spinach, and coffee.

Take vitamins and supplements. Although there is no definitive evidence that vitamins provide value in improving brain health, there are certain popular vitamins that people and some doctors believe aid the brain: vitamins E, B6, B12, C, and D, as well as omega-3 fatty acids.

Rest. Older people need between seven and nine hours of sleep. Inadequate sleep raises the risk for memory loss.

Maintain body function health. Heart problems, high blood pressure, high cholesterol, and diabetes, are all linked to poor brain health.

Treat depression. Depression doubles the risk for cognitive decline and dementia.

Treat hearing loss. A Johns Hopkins study found that older adults with hearing problems appear to have a greater rate of brain shrinkage as they age.

Avoid certain medications. Anticholinergic drugs have been shown to increase the risk of dementia. These drugs include antihistamines (Benadryl), sleep meds like Tylenol PM, and some antidepressants.

Treat stress. Stress and anxiety may cause memory problems, and longer-term stress is connected with faster rates of decline in brain health.

Play brain games and other cognitive exercises. Playing games and solving puzzles are excellent ways for older people to keep their brains active and alert. These activities stimulate the brain cells and often provide interaction with others.

Medications. Although, I would be skeptical about the effectiveness of medications in treating dementia, it may well be worth investigating medications as a form of treatment to help with cognitive symptoms, and some noncognitive symptoms such as mood and behavior. Check with your doctor for a list.

Coping with Dementia

Some coping skills are effective during the early stages of dementia. At first, memory loss creates awkward yet entertaining moments: "Where did my keys go?" After locating the keys during a 5-minute search, you may shrug off the temporary memory loss as harmless.

As memory loss worsens, it creates embarrassment and a loss of self-esteem for many people. Two coping skills have helped me deal with memory loss: acceptance and lifestyle change.

THE A'S HAVE IT

Acceptance. Acceptance is key for stress-free dementia. Accept your fate; memory loss is a permanent part of your life now. View memory loss and the early signs of dementia in a positive and possibly humorous light rather than as negative events.

Lifestyle changes. Organized people live less stressful lives than people who are disorganized, and this is especially true for people experiencing serious memory loss. Follow daily routines and do less multitasking. Strive to simplify your life wherever possible.

Unfortunately, most coping skills are ineffective for those dealing with late-stage dementia because of the significant loss in intellectual abilities like judgment and thinking, talking, learning, and reading. As their minds further deteriorate, severe physical problems like mobility loss, incontinence, and general frailty develop. People living alone with late-stage dementia won't survive long. They need assistance, including medical care or nurses and a social support network of family and friends.

Dementia can be sweet and sad at the same time. It is said that dementia is a condition that affects the brain but breaks the heart. Dementia attacks the spirit by weakening the mind's ability to reach the spirit. And as we know, people with dementia live in their own reality and are unable to fully comprehend the world around them. Some people with dementia are angry, some are paranoid, but some are also sweet and innocent. We all have stories about people with dementia.

There was a lady with dementia at the assisted living facility where my grandmother resided years ago. I remember her saying: "I'm 79, my mom's 79, and my grandma is 79! Isn't that funny?"

Dementia is perhaps the most difficult of all the inconveniences of aging, particularly for the family and close friends of the inflicted person. At present, there is little we can do to cure this affliction; all we can do is control it to a point. Possessing a sense of humor is a necessary component for all involved.

Age-Induced Depression

Physical or mental decline can result in serious consequences, triggering depression, helplessness, and a retreat from social activities, to name a few. This is the exception, not the rule. Most older adults can adequately cope with aging and find themselves in either the positive aging bucket or the practical aging bucket. However, some of us experience what I call age-induced depression and may find themselves confined to God's Waiting Room. It takes a special set of coping skills to avoid or minimize this depressed state.

When we are young, we are filled with hope and excitement about life. There is a beginning with no end. There are challenges and choices of what we want to do and what we want to be. Life is fresh and innocent as we begin our journey.

The journeys we embark on are as varied as the colors of the rainbow, but there is a common thread. Whether we choose to be teachers, construction workers, lawyers, or doctors, we all travel through a life cycle. Most of us experience childhood, attend school, marry, raise a family, work, and retire. We all participate in the game of life and discover, learn, and ponder. We experience happiness, sadness, hate, and love. No matter what each of us ends up doing in our lives, we will have lived a dynamic and robust reality.

Causes of Depression

At some point in our journey, hope dissipates, freshness goes stale, challenges become less meaningful, and the beginning approaches the end. For many of us, this is an inflection point in our lives. We transition from a dynamic, hope-filled life to a more stagnant, less meaningful existence. To survive, many of us can manage and revise our expectations of what life has to offer. We adjust to the fact that life is winding down and settle for simpler pleasures and challenges.

But for some of us, the dramatic shift to growing old from youthfulness is emotionally draining, resulting in sadness and perhaps depression. It is akin to postpartum depression, which is a mood disorder that can affect women after childbirth. A mother with postpartum depression experiences feelings of extreme sadness and anxiety that might interfere with her ability to care for herself or her family.

Age-induced depression is the realization that you have parted from your youthful years and are now aging and growing old. It can seem that we went from a dynamic and robust life to a more mundane existence in the blink of an eye—and some of us can't handle it. One day you are part of the action, and the next day you are standing on the sidelines watching the parade go by.

Although I did not experience age-induced depression, I can relate to people who do encounter the condition. As chief economist for some of the largest real estate associations in the nation, I was part of the intoxicating business and political world for many years. I appeared on or in major media like CNN, CNBC, the *Wall Street Journal*, and the *New York Times*, giving speeches across the nation and testifying before Congressional committees and working with the executive and legislative branches of government. And now I stand on the sidelines retired, watching others younger than me experience the fun and excitement of my previous life. It is not easy to no longer be invited to the party.

Sometimes the reality of life after work (retirement) doesn't live up to its promise. Upon retirement, we look forward to finally being able to focus on the things that give us greatest pleasure. Yet, according to a study by the London-based Institute of Economic Affairs,[26] The likelihood that someone will suffer from clinical depression goes up by about 40 percent after retiring. In large part that's because work, whether we realize it or not, provides many of the ingredients that fuel happiness, including social connections, a steady routine, and a sense of purpose.

Age-induced depression can be triggered by a midlife crisis or by retirement, or it could be triggered anytime that a person realizes that his or her life has less meaning than it once had. Again, similar to postpartum depression, which only some women experience, only a subset of older adults experience age-induced depression.

Symptoms of Depression

Symptoms of age-induced depression are plentiful for those who possess it. Feelings of sadness, hopelessness, and emptiness are common. Heightened anxiety and an indifference in making decisions could also occur. Societal isolation due to withdrawing from or avoiding friends, as well as suicidal thoughts, could also accompany this condition.

Obviously, someone experiencing age-induced depression has a more difficult time coping with the marks of aging. The key is to stay positive as we transition from a youthful, robust life to an aging, simple life. There are positive aging activities and remedies that we can do to help us avoid or minimize depression.

Ways to Manage and Lessen Depression

Please note: If you are experiencing severe depression, you need to see a medical professional.

Socialize. In the workforce, we enjoy established social relationships that diminish in retirement. Maintaining relationships post-retirement is important to your emotional well-being.

Maintain structure in your life. During the first half of our lives, we have some sort of structure and organization. We have a job to go to, a family to raise, etc. In the second half of life, particularly after retirement, our slate is pretty much blank. We need to provide structure in our lives, lined with tasks. Adhering to a routine helps you maintain a sense of purpose.

Acceptance and Affirmations. Affirmations like "I am great and accept myself as I age" might help you avoid a depressed state.

Continue employment. Some of us need to work, even in retirement, in order to lead a satisfying life. Part-time employment for retirees has increased in popularity.

Community service. Helping others is usually a good remedy to feel good about yourself. There is an abundance of community service opportunities in virtually every town in America.

Continuing education. One of the best ways to stimulate your mind and safeguard against depression is by continuing to learn as an older adult. That is why many sign up for college courses, often in subjects far afield from their former career.

These are just a few suggested remedies and activities to avoid age-induced depression. These and other positive aging activities are discussed in greater detail in chapter 13, Reclaim Your Life. The bottom line is that the second half of your life should be a joyful time, free of many of the responsibilities of your youthful working years. But you have to work to make it so.

Declining Mobility

The loss of mobility might be the most humbling of the inconveniences of aging. It is hard not to be shocked when you visit a senior living community and see so many residents using mobility devices. You can hear the walkers and rollators squeak and the wheelchairs and mobility scooters hum as residents march single file into the dining room. It's as if you've entered a war zone harboring wounded soldiers.

Many seniors with mobility issues postpone using canes, walkers, and rollators for fear of appearing old and helpless, even though these products improve quality of life. There is no shame in mobility loss—it's part of life. Canes, walkers, rollators, wheelchairs, and mobility scooters are cool; they improve quality of life.

Mobility is something people take for granted until they lose it. Just a twist of an ankle or a sharp pain in my foot throws me off for the whole day. Simple tasks like walking across a room, going to the bathroom, or getting out of bed or out of a chair can become difficult chores.

For many older people, loss of mobility turns their world inside-out because mobility loss has profound social and emotional consequences. Shopping or dinner with friends, for example, becomes overwhelming. People with serious mobility issues can become increasingly dependent on other people, which may result in depression and in some cases social isolation.

Aging causes many physical breakdowns in older people that contribute to mobility problems, including muscle weakness, joint problems, pain, disease, and neurological issue. Not surprisingly, the most common cause of mobility loss is falls. Falls causes broken bones and bruises that adversely affect mobility. Older bones break more easily than younger bones, and they heal less quickly and not as completely. If a hip is fractured, the need for canes, walkers, or wheelchairs might become permanent.

As we age, physical adroitness withers away. Some senior home residents wear scowls on their faces as they move about in their mobility devices, while others bravely smile. You can fight the aging war courageously with honor and pride or you can cower and retreat into self-pity. It's always been about the choices we make.

Treatments for Declining Mobility

Here are some ways to prevent or live with mobility problems:

Therapy. Physical therapy improves balance and strength training. Occupational therapy can help improve a person's ability to perform daily living activities and the living environment with tools such as elevated bathroom fixtures and grab bars.

Knee/Hip Replacement Surgery. If you continue to experience significant pain (due to arthritis) and mobility problems after a period of physical therapy, knee/hip replacement surgery is an option for many seniors. Soon canes and walkers for these specific cases could become a thing of the past.

Mobility Devices. The use of mobility devices such as canes, walkers, wheelchairs, and scooters assist people dealing with some mobility loss. They undeniably improve quality of life.

Canes

Canes are the first mobility product seniors turn to as they experience mobility issues. Some seniors postpone purchase of a cane due to the "old age" stigma associated with canes. Most manufacturers offer a limited variety of colors; canes are usually *made of* fiberglass or aluminum, although other lightweight *materials* such as graphite are now being used as well. Manufacturers are focused on producing ergonomic handles and height adjustability.

Walkers/Rollators

Rollators (three or four wheels) and walkers (no wheels or two wheels) are getting lighter and more functional and come in a variety of colors.

Wheelchairs and Mobility Scooters

There are manual and power wheelchairs and electric mobility scooters for people with mobility disabilities. Mobility scooters are the latest rage and will only increase in popularity as aging boomers involuntarily enter the market.

However, be sure you *need* a wheelchair or mobility scooter before you purchase one. My 95-year-old dad uses a walker and had been struggling to walk with one for some time. We told him to see a doctor and consider purchasing a mobility scooter so he could get around better in his senior center. To our surprise, the doctor recommended against using a mobility scooter. He said, that once my dad started using a mobility scooter, his muscles would atrophy, and he would no longer be able to walk again. He recommended physical therapy involving leg and knee exercises, as well as using a four-wheeled walker. It worked and my dad continues to walk—lessoned learned.

Exercise. Many different types of physical activity programs, ranging from simple home exercise programs to intensive, highly supervised hospital- or center-based programs, have been used to improve mobility in older people.

Coping with Declining Mobility

Loss of mobility diminishes quality of life, if you let it. How can you cope with mobility loss? One way is to employ the Four A's: accept, adapt, appreciate, and attitude.

THE A'S HAVE IT

Acceptance. You need to accept mobility decline if you are going to emotionally enjoy a quality life. Once you accept that you can no longer walk independently, you are set up for success. I remember that when my father was 88 years old he had a difficult time walking due to knee problems. His pride kept him from using a walker. Over the next year, he struggled mightily walking from room to room and to a table at restaurants. The day he gave in and used a walker was the day his quality of life improved.

Adaptation. Once you accept the reality of mobility loss, it's time to adapt. Fortunately, there are a host of mobility devices to facilitate a decline in mobility. As I stated previously, if your knees break, use a walker. If your eyes break, wear glasses. If your mind forgets, use a note reminder calendar. The sooner you use a cane, walker, or wheelchair, the sooner you are able to travel to places other than your chair and the sooner you will enjoy your life.

Attitude. Possessing the right attitude is key for coping with most inconveniences of aging, especially mobility decline. With the right attitude, you can learn to embrace mobility devices rather than disdain them. I know a gentleman at my parents' senior facility who shows off his mobility scooter. He rides the scooter around the building with a sense of pride.

It's out of our hands—mobility impairment happens to most of us as we age. The best we can do is to treat mobility devices as we treat automobiles. Have fun selecting the color and options and be proud of your new mode of transportation.

It's all about attitude when it comes to mobility problems and mobility devices. My friend Fast Eddie used a four-wheeled walker in his final years of life—(that's why we called him Fast Eddie). He had a great attitude and would say, "Mick Jagger has nothing on me—I can 'walk and roll' with the best of them."

Many people with mobility problems need assistance. It is hard enough to get into a car, but who is going to put the walker into the trunk? For people using walkers and wheelchairs, going to the bathroom is quite a task without help from others.

Hearing Impairment

More than any other inconvenience of aging, hearing loss requires that you maintain a sense of humor. A person with impaired hearing makes inappropriate remarks during conversations because he or she misheard the discussion, only to be the recipient of group laughter at his or her expense. We are embarrassed but try not to show it; maybe we even laugh along at ourselves.

More often than not, hearing loss is a gradual deterioration, so the impaired person may be in denial. This creates a difficult situation for all involved.

Fortunately, I haven't experienced serious hearing loss yet, but my 96-year old father has provided me with a boatload of stories and mixed emotions about the condition.

My dad says background noise makes it difficult to hear a person talking to him. He also has difficulty following a conversation when two or more people talk at the same time. Like most people with hearing loss, he admits to sometimes pretending to follow every word of a conversation that he has trouble following. He also nods and laughs a lot when people talk to him, hoping they don't ask him a question. People always seem to be mumbling their words. Sound familiar?

According to WebMD, about a third of Americans between the ages of 65 and 74 have hearing problems.[27] That statistic increases to 43 percent with age. Yet only one in five people who could benefit from a hearing aid actually wear one.

At 62, I'm showing signs of hearing loss. There are times when I ask my wife to repeat what she just said. I believe she speaks too softly now. I also have some trouble hearing clearly on a cell phone. These are common signs of hearing impairment; I will soon fall victim to serious hearing loss.

Like many baby boomers, I blame Led Zeppelin, The Who, and Bruce Springsteen for my current and future hearing woes. Boomers were the first generation exposed to loud music for hours at a time. My parents' generation listened to classical music, jazz, and Frank Sinatra, which are all soothing to the ear. Boomers were subjected to music blasted between 110 decibels (dB) and 120 dB, and maybe as high as 140 dB if you were in the front rows of a rock concert.

To demonstrate how loud a rock concert is, consider that normal talking is 40 dB to 60 dB. The softest sound that some humans can hear is 20 dB or lower. Headphones have a maximum volume set at 105 dB. I'm pretty sure Jimmy Page and Led Zeppelin took me beyond 140 dB on more than one occasion.

The human ear is like any other body part: aging and overuse can damage it. The inner part of the ear contains tiny hair cells (nerve endings). The hair cells change sound into electric signals. Then auditory nerves carry these signals to the brain, which recognizes them as sound. These tiny hair cells are easily damaged by loud sounds, particularly by repeated exposure to loud noise and music. This in turn can cause hearing loss.

Treatment of Hearing Impairment

Studies indicate that hearing impairment causes brain changes that increase the risk for dementia, making it especially important to treat your hearing loss in a timely manner. Here are some technology advancements we can use to improve hearing:

Hearing aids are electronic instruments you wear in or behind your ear. They make sounds louder. Ask for a trial period with your hearing aid and understand the terms and conditions of the trial period. Hearing aids can be expensive (in excess of $4,000) and your insurance company is likely not to cover the expense.

Cochlear implants are small electronic devices surgically implanted in the inner ear that help provide a sense of sound to people who are profoundly deaf or hard-of-hearing. If your hearing loss is severe, your doctor may recommend a cochlear implant in one or both ears.

Bone-anchored hearing systems bypass the ear canal and middle ear and are designed to use your body's natural ability to transfer sound through bone conduction. The sound processor picks up sound, converts it into vibrations, and then relays the vibrations through your skull bone to your inner ear.

Assistive listening devices include telephone and cell phone amplifying devices, smartphone or tablet apps, and closed-circuit systems (hearing loop systems) in places of worship, theaters, and auditoriums.

Coping with Hearing Impairment

Coping with hearing impairment is like coping with mobility decline—we need to deal with our ego's embarrassment about our impairment.

Many people are stressed-out and anxious about hearing loss and the prospects of having to wear a hearing aid. Denial is usually an initial reaction. You must push your ego and its negativity aside and accept the fact that you are hearing impaired. Again, as with mobility loss, acceptance is key to coping with hearing impairment.

Don't take yourself too seriously when you are unable to hear well in a conversation with others. Finding humor in this type of situation helps ease the awkwardness. Laugh out loud at your hearing problems—because what else can you do?

Live in the present moment and stop yearning for the days when your hearing was excellent. Use every available technology to help you better cope with hearing impairment. Wearing a hearing aid may well be a lifestyle change that you need to embrace.

The thing about hearing loss is that no one can see it. Most people are so impatient they just assume that the person with hearing loss is being rude or slow. Your kids may be (unknowingly) impatient with you because they have easily communicated with you over the years when you were younger and now you've disrupted that communicative relationship.

My message for anyone experiencing hearing loss is to put quality of life ahead of stubborn pride. Take the plunge and wear a hearing aid. If you choose not to, there could be a downside. If you wait too long to get a hearing aid, you may lose the ability to hear certain sounds, and you may not recover it even once you get a hearing aid. It is better to get one early than to wait too long. If you are the type of person who doesn't want to listen to everyone you meet—just turn the aid off; it's that simple.

By age 75, 48 percent of men and 37 percent of women experience hearing impairment. It's cool to wear hearing aids. Celebrity singers like Ariana Grande wear earpieces all the time on stage. So get with the program!

Wrinkles

A wrinkled old man was not one of the things I wanted to be when I grew up. If pushed, I can deal with age spots, skin tags, and angiomas. But wrinkles? Maybe a few here or there. But I don't want to shrivel. I don't want my skin to dry up and wither.

This was my attitude several years ago before I embraced my new notions for aging. Today, I accept wrinkles as part of my journey in life. To me, wrinkles are a reminder of what I've accomplished and endured in life. And frankly, wrinkles are not as bad as they are made out to be.

As skin ages it loses elasticity and becomes drier and more lined and wrinkled. Some people wrinkle more than others as they age. The dry weather in Colorado creates more wrinkles than if residents lived in a more humid state. The low humidity and high ultraviolet levels (because of high altitude) in the Rocky Mountain State wreaks havoc on your skin.

People with lighter skin have a propensity to wrinkle more than people with darker skin. The color of your skin is highly correlated to wrinkling. This is the result of the varying degrees of pigment that people produce. Darker skin has larger pockets in skin cells known as melanosomes, which contain the sticky pigment melanin. In darker skin, the melanin is packed so tightly that it absorbs and scatters more light, which provides more protection from the sun's ultraviolet rays.

The onset of wrinkles presents a challenge for most people. For many of us, wrinkles are the one mark of aging that represents growing old more than any other mark, so it causes negative emotions, such as anguish, sadness, and envy. How do we turn this negative energy into positive energy?

The good news is that superficial appearances matter less as you grow older, so wrinkles become less of an annoyance over time. Of course, your objective is to accept wrinkles earlier in your senior years, because you will lessen the stress and anguish usually associated with appearance deterioration. However, there is nothing wrong with taking steps to diminish or eliminate wrinkles to improve your appearance if you do it for the right reasons.

THE A'S HAVE IT

Adaptation. Alter your lifestyle to accommodate your older physical appearance. For example, don't let your ego convince you that you should try to look like a 30-year-old when you are 70. Doing this would only feed your ego with envy and other negativity.

Instead, try changing your hairstyle to better fit your age, wearing clothes that better compliment your mature look, and changing your makeup to better fit with your older face.

Attitude. Don't ever be ashamed about growing old, about your wrinkles, your age spots, or your other marks of aging. It's cool to be an older person. Attitude is everything!

Treatments for Wrinkles

Many baby boomers with a forever-young mindset spend billions of dollars every year on wrinkle creams, Botox, and plastic surgery. According to Transparency Market Research (transparencymarket-research.com), the antiaging product market was estimated to be worth $191 billion in 2019.

A good face lift might last eight to ten years, while facial fillers might last one to two years, and Botox will last about three months. Some of these treatments are not very effective, but people keep trying them.

No treatments have been rigorously shown to reverse aging. The biological process treks on underneath a veneer built on antiaging surgeries, applications, and creams. If you are contemplating plastic surgery, understand the risks. Plastic surgery sometimes works, but it can also go very wrong. But there is nothing wrong with wanting to diminish your wrinkled appearance as long as it is your spirit rather than your ego doing battle.

Fortunately, there are a number of treatments that are partially effective in preventing, diminishing, or eliminating (at least temporarily) wrinkles:

Avoid the sun or wear sunscreen. The sun's rays are the most cited cause of wrinkles.

Stop smoking. More studies are confirming that cigarette smoke ages skin by releasing an enzyme that breaks down collagen and elastin, which are two important components of the skin.

Antioxidants. These include vitamin A, C, and E, as well as beta-carotene. Products that have antioxidants may provide some sun protection and might mildly improve wrinkles. Fruits and vegetables are good sources of antioxidants.

Moisturizers. Moist skin has a healthier appearance, so wrinkles look less noticeable. But they don't make those lines go away permanently.

Omega-3 fatty acids. Consume more fish like salmon, which is a source of protein and omega-3 fatty acids that help nourish skin and may help to reduce wrinkles.

Skin care treatments. A variety of skin creams and other applications contain ingredients that may reduce wrinkles, including alpha-hydroxy acids, retinoids, topical vitamin C, Idebenone, and pentapeptides.

For those of you who want to battle wrinkles over the next decade or two, new medical technologies and innovations are available to diminish or eliminate wrinkles, including injections, wrinkle fillers, laser light resurfacing, chemical peels, dermabrasion, and plastic surgery.

Coping with Wrinkles

Battle wrinkles if it makes you feel healthy and alive. But do not mistake wrinkles with ugliness. Be proud of your wrinkles, not embarrassed.

Acceptance of your wrinkles occurs at some point in your life, usually around 70 or 80 years old. Remember, coping with wrinkles is really all about the ego. To disarm the ego, you must summon and strengthen your spirit. If you follow some of the ways presented in this book to tap into your spirit, you will soon appreciate that you are more than your physical body. Once this realization occurs, wrinkles are no longer a burden in your life.

Just like the rest of us, celebrities, too, have to cope with wrinkles. While many may use plastic surgery to cope, numerous celebrities have refused to go under the knife and have chosen to age gracefully instead. Many prominent celebrities are on record embracing wrinkles and wanting to destigmatize growing older.[28] Here are just a few:

Helen Mirren (73)
Diane Keaton (72)
Cameron Diaz (46)
Jamie Lee Curtis (59)
Reese Witherspoon (42)
Diane Von Furstenberg (71)
Drew Barrymore (43)

"Your face tells a story and it shouldn't be about your drive to the doctor's office."—Julia Roberts[29]

It is your choice whether you do anything about wrinkles, and if so, how much you are prepared to do. People who have taken care of themselves through natural remedies like a healthy diet, exercise, and positive lifestyle choices create not only a healthier appearance, but a self-confidence that helps them deal with the inevitability of aging.

American author Clarence Day once said: "Age should not have its face lifted, but it should rather teach the world to admire wrinkles as the etchings of experience and the firm line of character."

Your wrinkled face is a work of art that took years to create. Be proud to display it.

Coronavirus Pandemic

Confronting an epidemic/pandemic associated with a harmful or deadly disease is possibly the most disconcerting situation for an older person to face. As we age, our immune systems weaken, making us more vulnerable to the harmful effects of viruses and diseases. Moreover, many older persons already have pre-existing conditions (e.g., diabetes, cancer, and heart, lung, and immunological conditions) which make them even more at risk for contracting a potentially deadly virus/disease. It is no wonder that many older people respond to an epidemic/pandemic with heightened anxiety, and sometimes depression.

An epidemic is defined as an outbreak of a disease that occurs over a wide geographic area and affects an exceptionally high proportion of the population, while a pandemic is used to describe a disease that affects a whole country and/or the world.

As of this writing, the world is immersed in a serious pandemic: the coronavirus, or more specifically, COVID-19. From a historical perspective, today's coronavirus is the most recent in a long list of viruses and plagues that different parts of the world have dealt with over the centuries.

Here are the twenty worst epidemics and pandemics in history, including today's coronavirus.[30]

Plague of Athens:	430 B.C.
Antonine Plague:	165-180 A.D.
Plague of Cyprian:	250-271
(Bubonic) Plague of Justinian:	541-542
The Black Death:	1346-1353
Cocoliztli Epidemic:	1545-1548
American Plagues:	16th Century

Great Plague of London:	1665-1666
Great Plague of Marseille:	1720-1723
Russian Plague:	1770-1772
Philadelphia Yellow Fever Epidemic:	1793
Flu Pandemic:	1889-1890
American Polio Epidemic:	1916
Spanish Flu:	1918-1920
Asian Flu:	1957-1958
AIDs Epidemic:	1981-present
H1N1 Swine Flu Pandemic:	2009-2010
West African Ebola Epidemic:	2014-2016
Zika Virus Epidemic:	2015-present
Coronavirus (COVID-19):	2019-present

Coronavirus: COVID-19

According to the Mayo Clinic, coronaviruses are a family of viruses that can cause illnesses such as the common cold, severe acute respiratory syndrome (SARS), and Middle East respiratory syndrome (MERS). A new coronavirus was identified as the cause of a disease outbreak that originated in Wuhan, China, at the end of 2019. This virus is known as the severe acute respiratory syndrome coronavirus 2 (SARS-CoV-2), and it causes the coronavirus disease 2019, better known as COVID-19.

COVID-19, which began as an epidemic, is now a pandemic and has spread to more than 200 countries and territories as of this writing. The origins of this virus are thought to be evolutionary, not laboratory made. It likely jumped from an animal (probably a bat, although scientists are not completely certain) to a human.

The outbreak of COVID-19 is globally widespread because the virus is new, so people's immune systems are not prepared to fight it, permitting the virus to spread rapidly from person to person.

Our fight against this pandemic crisis is temporarily reshaping how we work and live. Millions of Americans are quarantining in their homes, most businesses have come to a grinding halt, all sporting and entertainment events are canceled, and hospitals are dealing with supply shortages of testing kits, swabs, and ventilators. The U.S. economy has fallen into a sharp recession with millions of people becoming unemployed, while the U.S. equities markets have plummeted, severely lowering the value of people's retirement portfolios.

Symptoms

The symptoms of COVID-19 appear two to fourteen days after exposure. They may include:

➢ Fever
➢ Cough
➢ Shortness of breath or difficulty breathing
➢ Fatigue
➢ Aches
➢ Runny nose
➢ Sore throat

Some people are asymptomatic but have contracted the virus. These people could unknowingly spread the virus to other people. The infection could be mild to some people, but it can also cause severe respiratory (or lung) illness in others and may result in death. It may also cause complications such as pneumonia or bronchitis. Severe complications or even death are more common with the elderly as well as people with a suppressed immune system or an underlying heart or lung disease. It is noted that a large study in China found that about 80 percent of confirmed cases of the virus had fairly mild symptoms. Unfortunately, about 15 percent of confirmed cases had experienced severe symptoms that caused significant shortness of breath, low blood oxygen, or other lung problems. About 5 percent of confirmed cases were critical, highlighted by respiratory failure, septic shock, or multiple organ problems.

According to the Center for Disease Control (CDC), those who are at high risk of contracting the virus include:

➤ Healthcare workers (and their close contacts) caring for people with COVID-19
➤ People returning from international destinations where community spread of the virus is occurring (China, Iran, South Korea, and Italy)
➤ People socializing in communities where community spread is active. Community spread means spread of the virus for which the source of infection is unknown.

COVID-19 appears to have a higher mortality rate than common illnesses such as seasonal flu. The World Health Organization's director general, Dr. Tedros Adhanom Ghebreyesus, has speculated a mortality rate of 3.4 percent. But because there are probably many more people with the virus who go undetected, the mortality rate is likely closer to 1 percent, which is still ten times greater than the 0.1 percent mortality rate of most flus.

The combination of how quickly and easily the coronavirus can spread and the severity of the illness has prompted many nations (including America), to take drastic public health measures to contain and limit the impact of the pandemic. At one point, virtually all "nonessential" Americans had been asked to stay home in an effort to curb the coronavirus pandemic.

As of this writing, there is no cure for COVID-19, but efforts to develop a vaccine for COVID-19 are on the front burner for scientists around the world. A number of scientific teams are already testing vaccine candidates in animals and preparing to carry out trials on people. It may take twelve to eighteen months for an effective vaccine against COVID-19 to be readily available to the public.

Avoidance and Treatment

In any epidemic or pandemic, there are always government guidelines for avoidance. For COVID-19, avoidance guidelines are straightforward:

- ➢ Wash hands thoroughly with soap and water for twenty seconds
- ➢ Practice social distancing: stand six feet apart from other people
- ➢ No crowds with more than ten people
- ➢ Stay home
- ➢ Wear a mask when out

For people who begin to show symptoms of the virus, there are several things they can do to treat their immediate health problem. First, stay home for at least fourteen days, keeping away from other people. Second, take your temperature regularly throughout the day. Third, take an acetaminophen like Tylenol to reduce fever. Fourth, call a healthcare professional if the symptoms persist. And finally, go to the nearest test site for testing.

Coping with the Threat of Coronavirus (COVID-19)

The coronavirus spreads fear, isolation, and possibly death to older adults. In some cases, the virus is a personal nightmare for people with anxiety and depression. We are living in a stressful time, so it is particularly important for older people to take care of their mental health. Practicing positive aging has never been more important for older people than coping with today's coronavirus pandemic.

Here are some ways to cope:

Strengthen your ability to fight the virus. Senior citizens are more vulnerable to COVID-19 because people's immune systems weaken with age. Although there are no immunity silver bullets, it is important that older people make sure they are not deficient in certain nutrients. This is because without enough of the essential nutrients your body needs, your immune system suffers. For example, many studies show that deficiencies in vitamins C and D are frequently found in people with infections, including pneumonia.

The best way of assuring that your body is getting a sufficient amount of vitamins, minerals, and other nutrients is to eat a wide variety of foods. A diet rich in antioxidants (vitamins A, C, and E) plus vitamin D, zinc, and selenium should help maintain a healthy immune system as we age.

> - Vitamin A: Squash, carrots, spinach, sweet potatoes, dark leafy greens
> - Vitamin C: Citrus fruits, broccoli, tomatoes, strawberries
> - Vitamin E: Almonds, wheat germ, whole grains
> - Vitamin D: tuna, salmon, beef liver, cheese, egg yolks
> - Zinc: nuts, dairy, shellfish, legumes (lentils, chickpeas)
> - Selenium: Oysters, halibut, eggs, sunflower seeds, chicken breasts

Of course, if you are unable to consume a wide variety of foods in your diet, you may supplement your diet with the appropriate vitamin and mineral tablets.

Exercise. There is no substitute for staying healthy and fit when preparing to fight off a flu or virus. Moderate exercises include walking (at least 5,000 steps or more per day), jogging, gardening, light weightlifting, and yoga, all of which can be practiced as solo activities during a pandemic.

Get enough sleep. Getting the right amount of quality sleep aids your natural infection resistance. There is a link between sleep and a healthy immune system. For most adults, seven to eight hours of uninterrupted sleep is recommended. It would help if you limit or avoid consuming caffeine during this pandemic period.

Practice social isolation. Practicing social isolation is critical for the high-risk segment of the senior citizen population. My 91-year-old mother lives in an independent living facility and no outside person, including family, is permitted on the premises. Further, the building's dining room is closed, forcing all the residents to eat their meals alone in their respective apartments.

Isolation can trigger loneliness, anxiety and, possibly depression. Older people in isolation must maintain a positive mindset to maintain their mental health and well-being. Fortunately, there are ways to socially connect without physically connecting.

People can digitally connect via their smart phones and laptop computers. There are a host of online senior groups to chat with other seniors (Google "online senior chat groups"). You can also connect by telephone by calling the Institute on Aging's Friendship line. It's a hotline where older people can make a friend over the phone. And of course, family members of isolated seniors need to call them regularly.

Practicing isolation does not preclude you from taking long walks outside as long as you stay six feet away from others. Walking is a way to clear your mind of negative thoughts, tap into your spirit, and maintain a positive mindset.

Reduce anxiety and depression. Practicing mindfulness and positivity lessens the magnitude of your anxiety and depression about the coronavirus pandemic. Just reading or watching the daily news reports about the coronavirus can be anxiety-inducing. Staying in the present moment will lessen your anxiety about the future, including your fears about contracting the virus. Select an affirmation about positive things in your life and regular repeating it to help control your depressed thoughts. And more importantly, if you believe your heightened anxiety and/or depression is out of your control, do not be afraid to call a healthcare professional.

Calm fear and uncertainty. The coronavirus pandemic has injected fear and uncertainty into people's daily lives. The key is to avoid seeing yourself as the victim, because if you do, you will inevitably fall victim in today's pandemic environment. Rather than play victim, embrace the role of positivity and you will see yourself in a positive light even under the most trying conditions. And if you believe in the law of attraction, your positive thoughts will bring you only positive outcomes within a virus-worrisome environment. In the end, the coronavirus problem is not about the things that happen to us, but how we choose to respond to them. Practicing positivity keeps us in control of how we react to the events surrounding us.

Pray. Many people turn to their faith when facing troubled times. Prayer is a profound way to tap into your spirit and communicate with what some believe to be God, and what others believe to be a higher self. Either way, prayer is an effective way of emotionally surviving the potential ravages of the coronavirus pandemic. However, during the coronavirus pandemic, houses of worship are closed to the public to keep people from gathering in large crowds. For millions of people, not attending church on a Sunday (or Saturday for Jewish temples) is coronavirus's cruelest restriction.

So, you need to pray more in isolation. Summon your spirit and learn to stay in the present moment; this will help you maintain an effective solo prayer session. Of course, there are other ways to participate in group prayer without being physically present, such as online prayer groups and watching religious leaders lead people in prayer on television.

Coping with the COVID-19 Infection

If you contract the coronavirus, you will likely experience one or more of the symptoms most associated with the COVID-19 disease: fever, trouble breathing or shortness of breath, coughing, body aches, runny nose, tiredness, and sore throat. For most younger people without any pre-existing health conditions, these symptoms are modest and can be tolerated. However, for many older people and especially those with pre-existing heart, lung, and immunological conditions, these symptoms may inflict great harm and pain, and possibly death. Practicing three of the four A's—acceptance, appreciation, and attitude—will help you cope with your physical challenges.

THE A'S HAVE IT

Acceptance. Embracing acceptance helps you cope better with physical failings. Accepting the notion of having COVID-19 and that it will temporarily (hopefully) change your life, sets you up for success.

Appreciation. It is natural to embrace hopelessness when you are inflicted with the virus's symptoms, especially when you suspect these symptoms will get harsher and inflict greater pain. Embrace appreciation and you will see the good in every situation. You will be grateful for what your life was and appreciate your life in the present moment. Appreciate your life and you begin to love yourself. More importantly, appreciation gives you the patience to endure whatever suffering you experience from the symptoms of the coronavirus.

Attitude. It goes without saying that possessing the right attitude is key for coping with COVID-19 symptoms, as well as coping with an eventual serious illness. Don't cower to the fear and uncertainty that the virus inflicts on our emotions. And if the virus becomes life-threatening, a positive attitude becomes critical for maintaining your mental health, let alone your survival.

Facing prospects of death. For older people, especially those with pre-existing conditions, contracting COVID-19 introduces the fear of dying into a person's life. Coping with your awareness of mortality is not easy. Aside from leaning on religious prayer and other supernatural beliefs, it might help to lean on the belief that you are more than your physical body by becoming more spiritual. You might find comfort in the belief that your spirit lives on after death. Do not live in fear of the prospects of death; instead, embrace every moment as if it were your last.

Final Thoughts

I chose to focus on how to live and cope with today's coronavirus pandemic because the pandemic may live on for at least another year or two after the release of this book. Hopefully, the worst will be over by the book's release date, but I have no way of knowing as of this writing.

None of us can return to the way we were before COVID-19. At the very least, seniors need to adapt their lifestyles to retool for this new normal. They need to navigate a disrupted world that is now less social. Until a vaccine is widespread, the novel coronavirus poses a risk of disease, especially to those over 65 years of age who are deemed high risk. Thus, seniors should take prudent steps (i.e., preventive measures) to reduce their risk of infection:

- Cover your mouth when you sneeze or cough
- Maintain good hand hygiene
- Replace handshakes with waves and air kisses, or elbow touching
- Regularly monitor temperature
- Be aware of symptoms
- Maintain a healthy immune system
- Wear face masks when appropriate (in large crowds)
- Exercise (e.g., walking)
- Stay connected (via video chat, online support groups, etc.)
- Avoid crowded restaurants, movie theaters, and events
- Practice meditation/mindfulness
- Maintain a positive mindset

The coronavirus pandemic dominates our lives today, and senior citizens are the demographic group in America most vulnerable to the harmful effects of the disease. Practicing positive aging by utilizing some of the tools, notions, and practices presented in the preceding chapters offers extraordinary assistance to help aging older adults survive what might become the most arduous health scare of their lives.

CHAPTER TEN

Aging to the Other Side

I believe aging consists of two phases. Phase I is the aging transition—the revelation that you are aging and declining. As you age, you are confronted with the harsh reality that you will never be the same, as you can plainly see after reading the list of diseases and illnesses and impairments in the previous chapter. Arthritis is a good example of a Phase I trigger event. The most common form, osteoarthritis, causes pain, swelling, and an overall lower quality of life for millions of older people. Arthritis is a wakeup call that you are growing old.

Phase II is the final transition, the revelation of mortality that can be triggered by any number of dire events. An event, such as being diagnosed with cancer or suffering a severe heart attack, is usually what opens the curtains of finality. The reality of mortality also surfaces for many older people who are confined to wheelchairs because of severe mobility decline. For some older people, a Phase II final transition results in lower self-worth, depression, and a declining passion for life.

Your coping skills for aging apply nicely to Phase I transitioning. Living in Phase II is a more difficult challenge but applying your coping skills will help here as well.

THE A'S HAVE IT

Appreciation. Appreciate that you are still present on Earth no matter what your physical appearance has morphed into. Life may not be as exciting or as passionate as it once was, but you can still smell the roses, feel the sun's rays, and savor the love of your children. There is a wonderful quote about life: "Life is not about how you survived the storm; it's about how you danced in the rain."

Some older people voluntarily step aside and let younger people pass because they believe it's the younger people's turn to experience the joys and sorrows of life. However, I believe there is room for all of us. We are not finished yet. Life is precious and we are going to honor and appreciate every moment of it. For aging baby boomers, we are entering the Third Act of our lives; there is still so much to do.

Phase I: Aging Transition

Perhaps you've heard the myth that the human body replaces itself every seven years or so. This myth asserts that we become essentially new people, because in that timespan every cell in our bodies has been replaced by a new cell. There are between 50 and 75 trillion cells in the human body and each has its own life span; cells die and are replaced continually, so there is nothing special about a seven-year cycle. But there is no denying that over time, our physical bodies age and deteriorate to a point where some of us become unrecognizable from our former (younger) selves.

The long process of transitioning into an older person is perhaps the greatest inconvenience of aging, even though it is not a specific physical or mental mark associated with growing old. The cumulative physical changes of aging are noticeable to all: wrinkles, shrinking, hair loss, hearing and vision impairment, reduced libido, and more. Older people, in effect, transition into different bodies. The fact that your general appearance changes so dramatically as you age is tough for many people to handle.

However, behind the altered physical veneer are the emotional transitions to a different way of life. Most people involuntarily downshift their lives as they age; they move from center stage to the sidelines. They transition from a dynamic life filled with hopes and dreams to a static life of retirement and reflection, and sometimes stagnation and helplessness. What was previously a vibrant, youthful existence can become a stale life filled with insecurities and doubt.

One day, you are young, healthy, independent, and unaware of your mortality, and the next day you experience declining health and find yourself frail and dependent upon others.

You can choose to age rather than live...and you will become an old fart. Or you can choose to forever age and live a joyous life in an older person's body. It's your choice. In this phase of aging, you get to choose whether you will spend your time hanging out in God's Waiting Room, the Practical Aging Room, or the Positive Aging Room.

I choose the latter, but that doesn't mean I'm not nervous about aging to the other side. In fact, I look for signs of aging before they even occur. I regularly inspect my skin for new age spots, signs of skin cancer, or new wrinkles. At first, for most of us, these marks arrive unannounced with little fanfare, as if they are embarrassed to show up. A slight graying at the temples or an age spot here or there. At some point the floodgates open and you transition from a middle-aged adult to an older person. Sometimes I feel as if my body is a time share: I have the same identity but in a different body.

If you are over 50 years old, how many of the high school yearbook pictures of your classmates can you match to their current pictures on Facebook? It is amazing how most of us physically transition to the "other" side of aging. It is also remarkable how time strikes people in different ways. The high school yearbook/Facebook exercise is not intended to poke fun at aging classmates—in fact, it is just the opposite. It's to demonstrate that over time, your physical appearance is irrelevant. The only change in these classmates is the way they look;

they remain the same people with the same personalities and spirits/ souls as before the transition.

Do any of us look like we did 30 or 40 years ago? Just look again at your Facebook friends from high school. Most of them are grandparents now and look the part, compared to their salad days of high school.

Actress Susan Sarandon said it best: "I look forward to being older, when what you look like becomes less and less an issue and what you *are* is the point."[31]

Ways to Ease the Aging Transition

Many of us get emotionally lost in transition. Emotional and social changes prove to be difficult and troubling. Many older people become lonely and have fewer meaningful things in their lives as they transition. Some of us move into God's Waiting Room without even making visits to the Positive Aging Room or even the Practical Aging Room. I easily could have moved into God's Waiting Room after my cancer diagnosis.

It doesn't have to be this way. In fact, there are a great many older people who successfully make the transition to the aging transition phase. There is no set formula for how to accomplish this. You may place greater emphasis on some notions and practices of aging and less emphasis on others, depending on your physical and mental strengths and weaknesses.

The objective is to make the changes needed to achieve a more balanced life, so you can cope with aging to the other side. Consider the actions listed below as initial food for thought. Also, review the practices discussed in chapters 3 through 8 and in the next few chapters to discover more ideas about optimizing your body, mind, emotions, and inner spirit so that you can enjoy more days in the Positive Aging Room.

Take Advantage of Technology

I implore you to make use of all available technology as you age to the other side. If you have mobility problems, use a walker. If you have hearing impairment, wear a hearing aid. If you have heart problems, replace a valve or undergo a heart transplant.

Do whatever it takes. Knee replacement surgery is becoming commonplace for people with creaky knees. Within the next decade, there will be technology solutions and options for just about every body part. Stay medically and technically informed.

Strive for Balance

As discussed in chapter 8, balance is key in aging well. Unfortunately, just as we often begin to have problems with our physical balance as we age, so we often struggle with our life balance. Apply the notions you've read so far in this book in whatever combination and with whatever emphasis you choose—figure out what works for you! If you still feel stressed-out and negative, check to see if the elements in your life are balanced.

For example, how do you feel about having too many doctor visits every month? Are you taking too many medications? Are you regularly exercising? Are you on a healthy diet? Are you socializing with negative people?

You will know you have achieved balance when you regularly experience inner peace and live a joyous life in your senior years.

In 1971, a folk singer named John Prine wrote a song titled "Hello in There." Although Prine was only 25 years old when he wrote the song, he captured the loneliness older people experience when transitioning in aging. I find these lines particularly poignant:

Ya' know old trees just grow stronger
And old rivers grow wilder every day
Old people just grow lonesome
Waiting for someone to say, "Hello in there, hello."

Then there's the old saying "Don't judge a book by its cover," which especially applies to older people because there is a dynamic life history behind every one of them.

Older people want to be noticed and respected rather than shunned. Yesterday, our identities were shaped by how we raised our families, how we grew in our careers, and how we were involved in the community. This is all behind us now. Older people understandably struggle to maintain an identity in the uncertain world of aging.

Phase II: The Final Transition

Growing old is a picnic compared to the prospect of death. I know firsthand about cancer and mortality, and many of us have had similar brushes with death. However, the continuing advances of medical technology have altered attitudes toward dying. Dying is no longer part of human daily consciousness or an accepted final event of life. The famed psychiatrist Elizabeth Kubler-Ross insisted that the dying stage of life can be experienced as the most profound event in life. Dying begins when the facts of life are finally recognized, communicated, and accepted.

Dr. Kubler-Ross taught that there were five stages of grief in the dying phase of life:

➢ Denial
➢ Anger
➢ Bargaining
➢ Depression
➢ Acceptance

These states are not linear, and some people may not experience any of them. Others might only undergo one or several stages rather than all five.[32]

Older people (as well as those with life-threatening conditions) tend to think about dying and death more than any other age group. Most researchers consider the fear of dying as the most prevalent emotion for older people. Yet other emotions linked to death and dying can also be found in the mix, such as hope and feelings of loss (e.g., loss of control, competence, independence, people, or dreams for the future).

As a society, we have traditionally shied away from death and the idea of termination. But in recent years research has led people toward greater awareness and an increased interest in the dying process. Spirituality and storytelling can be used as resources in aging successfully and in dying, given the constraints of the modern-day western culture.

The fear of finality is where everyone freaks out. Most of us become, dare I say, irrational, perhaps even believing in tales told thousands of years ago by people who thought a flat Earth was the center of the universe. I call this madness over mortality; it's a special inconvenience of aging.

No one has definitive answers about humankind's relationship with the cosmos, so everyone is entitled to their own beliefs about life and the universe, as crazy as they may be. We all have a free pass to act as loony and foolish as we would like if that's what helps us deal with our mortality.

We live in a spiritual marketplace for coping with the inevitability of death. It is filled with supernatural products ranging from the traditional religions of Judaism, Christianity, and Islam to the Eastern religions/philosophies of Buddhism and Hinduism to the New Age beliefs such as the Law of Attraction, the Power of Now, astral travel, and various mystical beliefs. If you have faith in a spiritual paradigm, the remaining years of your life can become more bearable. People who have doubts are likely to become preoccupied with death in their senior years. They say things like, "What's the point? I'm going to die soon so why take on new challenges?" Obsessing over death is the most direct route to God's Waiting Room.

What drives me crazy is that this irrational behavior makes sense because we have few other options than to believe in an afterlife. Atheism isn't much of an option for me because, as some anonymous person once wrote, "It feels like I'm all dressed up and nowhere to go."

Did you know that your probability of dying during a given year doubles every eight years? British actuary Benjamin Gompertz first noticed this startling fact in 1825 and it is now called the Gompertz-Makeham law of mortality. If you are a 25-year-old, your probability of dying during the next year is a fairly minuscule .03 percent, or about 1 in 3,000. When you are 33, it will be about 1 in 1,500; when you are 42, it will be about 1 in 750. By the time you reach 100 year old, the probability of living to 101 will only be about 50 percent. This is a seriously rapid progression: Your mortality rate is increasing exponentially with age.

Coping with Mortality

Humans are quite different from other animals—we are aware of our own mortality, while lions, bears, and birds are not. So, how do people cope with awareness of finality? By creating beliefs and values that promise a sense of immortality.

Leave a social legacy. For many people, dying feels more digestible if you leave something meaningful behind when you pass away. For example, you get a piece of immortality if you climb to the peak of Mount Everest. Any achievement, whether it's in your community or in your business, gives you a piece of immortality.

Leave a family legacy. Most of us have children because if fulfills a need to leave a legacy—our biological children.

Find meaning in life. If you find meaning in life, you face death with your head held high because you probably do not consider your life wasted. Helping others through community service or joining the military are some ways that people find meaningfulness in their lives.

Religion and Mortality

Traditional religions. Becoming more religious and adopting supernatural beliefs is the easy way out of this mortality dilemma. A religion offering an afterlife brings purpose to this life. If you become religious and are convinced there is a heaven and God, you are immediately saved from the ugly hands of the Grim Reaper.

New Age beliefs. The Power of Now and the Law of Attraction are New Age beliefs that hold there is some energy force that keeps it altogether—that we are all part of something bigger. It gives you a taste of immortality.

Eastern religious beliefs. Most Eastern religions, like Buddhism, believe in reincarnation. When you die you come back to live another life, over and over again. Sounds like a good gig if you can get it.

THE A'S HAVE IT

Acceptance and Appreciation. If all you do with your life is worry about losing it, you might as well be dead. Live every moment on Earth as a gift. When I was a younger man, my best friend's dad died at age 53; it was a mortality wake-up call for us. We were only 17 at the time and were suddenly forced to realize that life was precious. Since then I stop often to watch the sun rise and set, flowers bloom, and birds sing. It sounds corny but it works for me. If you are not afraid to live, you will be less afraid to die.

Final Thoughts

Death is hereditary, so let's blame it on our parents.

Steve Jobs said it best: "No one wants to die. Even people who want to go to Heaven don't want to die to get there. And yet death is the destination we all share. No one has ever escaped it. And that is as it should be, because Death is very likely the single best invention of Life. It is Life's change agent. It clears out the old to make way for the new."[33]

Woody Allen quipped: "I'm not afraid of death—I just don't want to be there when it happens."[34]

I met a frail 87-year-old man who uses a four-wheel walker at a senior center in the town where I live. He looks helpless, lost, and unhappy. The manager of the center told me he sits in a chair in the lobby for hours, staring out the window and speaking to no one. The manager also told me that this lonely man was one of the leading scientists on the team that put man on the moon. He was also a professor at Stanford whose research was widely published in scholarly journals. He lived a fascinating life in his younger days, but you would never know it unless you asked.

Is this going to happen to you and me? How do we avoid getting lost in transition? Physically morphing into an old man or lady is little league compared to the emotional transition of living life in our waning years.

I've come to believe aging is both a blessing and a curse. Physical deterioration is a curse, but with aging comes spiritual growth, which is a blessing. As older adults, we need to focus on our spirits, not our bodies.

An old girlfriend once told me, "Nobody cares if you can't dance. Just get up and dance." This same attitude is what being a senior citizen and growing old is about. There is no need to be embarrassed that you are old, and you shouldn't stop doing things because you can no longer do them well. Just do them until you can't anymore!

CHAPTER ELEVEN

Healthy Habits for Your Body

We can't bypass the aging process, but we *can* avoid aging too quickly. So, why not be proactive and take steps to avoid the pitfalls that could accelerate the aging process? A successful positive aging path includes addressing the health of your body and your emotions. Even as you confront the inconveniences of aging and accept the inevitable changes, you can still practice healthy habits and maintain healthy nutrition to meet the needs of an aging physical body.

Healthy Habits

Here are some good suggestions to keep your body as healthy as possible.

Simplify Your Life

Staying too busy can be stressful. Trying to complete an endless list of doctor appointments, errands, visiting grandkids, and socializing with friends can be overwhelming. Chronic stress triggers the release of cortisol into your bloodstream. Cortisol causes an increase in your heart rate and blood pressure. Keeping life simple and stress-free helps prevent aging too quickly.

Maintain a Healthy Weight

Maintaining a healthy weight is important for your overall well-being. If you are too heavy, you run the risk of heart disease, stroke, diabetes, and high blood pressure.

Exercise

Regular exercise yields many health benefits, including having more energy, feeling happier, strengthening your muscles and bones, and reducing your risk of chronic disease, to name just a few. For some older people, exercise includes lifting weights as well as aerobics (e.g., briskly walking)

Get Enough Sleep

Insufficient sleep on a nightly basis is associated with a greater risk of health problems (e.g., diabetes), which obviously are more critical as you grow older.

Keep Structure in Your Life

For some people, retirement means a less-structured life compared to the structure of a regular 9 to 5 jobs. Having little structure in your life can result in a directionless existence that brings with it its own set of emotional issues. Working part-time is a good option, but if you don't want to work you need to find some forms of structure in your life. Put yourself on a schedule: wake up at the same time every morning, go for a walk, exercise, read, volunteer at community centers, and so forth.

Practice Proper Posture

This is something that never occurred to me—but I recently read that poor posture can be harmful to your health as you age. This is because poor posture deviates the spine from normal alignment, which results in abnormal stress on muscles, disks, and bones. Poor posture is a primary contributor to pain and fatigue in older adults. Good posture involves training your body to stand, walk, and sit in positions where the least strain is placed on supporting muscles, ligaments, and bones.

Stop Sitting All the Time

Staying in a sedentary position for a prolonged period of time—like when you sit on a couch for hours binge-watching television—is an unhealthy activity (or should I say, *in*activity). People who are sedentary are at risk for kidney disease and cardiovascular disease—not to mention obesity.

Visit Professional Health Practitioners Regularly

Visiting doctors regularly and making sure you are getting the right nutrition in your meals and supplement with vitamins are steps in the right direction. You should be getting plenty of iron, omega-3 fatty acids, calcium, and vitamin D in your diet, as well as B12 and potassium (see Healthy Nutrition, below). You also need to monitor your blood pressure and cholesterol levels, and examine your skin on a regular basis, looking out for any unusual tags, moles, etc.

Healthy Nutrition

According to Susan Landeis, CNC (certified nutritional consultant),[34] focusing on changing nutritional needs is a crucial step in managing senior citizen health and well-being as we age. It is obvious that our nutritional needs change as we age. Here are some of her reasons why:

➤ Seniors become less mobile and lose muscle

➤ Metabolic rates decrease with age, requiring fewer needed calories

➤ Poor teeth/dentures make it more difficult to eat solid foods

➤ Swallowing problems also make it difficult to eat solid foods

➤ Diminished taste/smell/eyesight could result in less enthusiasm for certain foods

➤ Gastrointestinal changes may result in avoidance of healthy foods

➤ Social isolation may lead to an indifference toward eating healthy meals

➤ Memory loss or other cognitive issues may result in forgetting to eat

Aside from the medical benefits, maintaining a healthy nutritional diet raises energy levels and minimizes sadness and depression. Landeis identifies the most common nutritional deficiencies in seniors as they age:

➤ Vitamin A, B (especially B12), C, D, and E

➤ Calcium

➤ Fiber

➤ Protein

➤ Potassium

➤ Magnesium

➤ Zinc

Get Your Vitamins

Maintaining appropriate levels of vitamin B is particularly important for aging seniors. Vitamin B12 deficiency can cause severe nerve and brain damage.[35] Folic acid is another vitamin B that helps protect against heart disease and cancer.

Vitamin D is also important for bone strength, nerve function, and calcium absorption. If you are calcium deficient, you may be at risk for osteoporosis and fragile bones. Women and people with darker complexions tend to have a higher risk of vitamin D deficiency than men and people with light complexions.

Vitamin D is made by our bodies in the skin when we are exposed to sunlight. Older skin is not as efficient at producing vitamin D, and older adults can be especially at risk because they don't get outside as much. Vitamin D is important for bone strength, nerve function, and calcium absorption. If you are not getting enough calcium, you may be at risk for osteoporosis, fragile bones, and falling. Calcium comes from dairy products or calcium supplements.

Women tend to have a higher risk than men for vitamin D deficiency, and people with darker complexions don't produce vitamin D as well as people with lighter complexions. Also know that certain drugs such as steroids, cholesterol-lowering drugs, acid-reducing meds, and weight loss drugs can all interfere with vitamin D supplements. The best food sources for vitamin D are salmon, tuna, cheese, egg yolks, beef liver, cereal, milk, and juice.

The best sources for fiber are apples, berries, squash, and many other fruits and vegetables. Fiber improves digestion and helps lower cholesterol and maintain blood sugar levels.

Foods such as white beans, yogurt, bananas, broccoli, and red peppers contain calcium, magnesium, and potassium, which helps lower blood pressure.

CHAPTER TWELVE

Emotional Intelligence and Aging

In my search for ways to cope with aging, I noticed how the traits contributing to a person's emotional intelligence intersect with the positive aging practices (i.e., spirit, mindfulness, positivity, the Four A's, social support, and balancing) presented in this book. It may be worthwhile to take a closer look into emotional intelligence and how it may elevate our ability to cope with aging.

Wikipedia defines emotional intelligence, or EI, as the capability of individuals to recognize their own emotions and those of others, discern between different feelings and label them appropriately, use emotional information to guide thinking and behavior, and manage or adjust emotions to adapt to environments or achieve one's goals.[36]

Today, EI is applied to the workplace. Many employers are realizing that the key to building a successful team begins with understanding and developing the EI of their employees. EI has proved to be a strong indicator of worker performance, development potential, and an employee's ability to work effectively with others.

For seniors, having emotional intelligence is essential for successful aging. After all, who is more likely to succeed, a senior citizen who is anxious, stressed-out, and sometimes depressed, or a senior who stays calm under stress and stays in control even under the onslaught of the marks of aging.

For our purposes, emotional intelligence is presented in five broad categories as defined by the coaching and human development company Upward Solutions.[37]

- ➤ Self-Perception
- ➤ Stress Management
- ➤ Decision-Making
- ➤ Self-Expression
- ➤ Interpersonal

The more that you, as a senior citizen aging, manage and develop each of the five elements of EI presented here, the greater the likelihood that you will age successfully. Let's look at each element in more detail and examine how you can grow your EI. Our approach is to apply EI to the business of aging rather than leading a staff of workers.

Self-Perception

Self-perception involves several components, including self-regard and self-actualization. A third component is self-awareness. If you're self-aware, you always know how you feel, you understand your emotions, and you know how your emotions and your actions can affect your ability to cope with physical and mental decline. You possess the ability to differentiate between subtleties in your own emotions while understanding the cause(s) of these emotions and the impact they have on your thoughts and actions and those of others around you, including family and caregivers.

Being self-aware when you are aging also means understanding and accepting one's strengths and weaknesses, which is very much tied to life balancing (chapter 8). Seniors with a healthy self-perception will likely try to improve themselves by adapting to the physical and mental changes they experience as they age.

Here are some ways to improve your self-perception:

Keep a journal. Journals help you improve your self-awareness. Just a few minutes each day writing down your thoughts can move you to a higher degree of self-awareness.

Slow down. When you experience anger or other strong emotions, slow down to examine why. Remember, no matter what the situation, you can always choose how you react to it.

Meditate. Meditation is another way to slow down and calm yourself. Meditate for just a few minutes a day and you will become more self-aware. (See chapters 3, The Power of Me: Inner Spirit, and 5, Positivity, for more on this subject.)

See the big picture. Go 10,000 feet in the air (figuratively) and look down at your situation. This gives you a macro view of your condition and life. It gives you a broader perspective of yourself.

Revisit your values. As seniors age, there are times when we become insecure about our lives; we lose self-esteem. Revisit your values and get to know your self-worth.

Stress Management

According to Dr Stephen Palmer, Director of the Centre for Stress Management in London, stress is the psychological, physiological, and behavioral response by an individual when they perceive a lack of equilibrium between the demands placed upon them and their ability to meet those demands—which, over a period of time, leads to ill-health.[38]

To manage stress, we need to adapt emotions, thoughts, and behaviors to unfamiliar, unpredictable, and dynamic circumstances. For seniors coping with stressful physical and mental decline, we need to believe that we can manage or influence these situations in a positive manner. In other words, we need to maintain optimism in a stressful situation.

Optimism is an indicator of one's positive attitude and outlook on life. It involves remaining hopeful and resilient, despite occasional setbacks. (See chapter 5: Positivity.)

Stress management is all about staying in control and avoiding rushed or emotional decisions. To some degree, it is about controlling your ego, which displays envy, anger, and frustration under stress. This element of emotional intelligence, according to author and researcher Daniel Goleman, also covers a senior's flexibility and commitment to personal accountability. Seniors who can self-regulate do not compromise their values, and they maintain their self-esteem even under dire circumstances.[39]

From a health perspective, stress is harmful and may contribute to cardiovascular disease, diabetes, and anxiety/depression.

Here are some ways to improve stress management:

Be accountable. Get hold of your ego. If you tend to blame the world or others when something goes wrong, stop. Make a commitment and accept your physical and mental decline and face the consequences, whatever they are.

Stay calm. The next time you are confronted with a mark of aging (e.g., hearing impairment) in a challenging situation, be aware of how you act. Do you relieve your stress by shouting at someone else or even yourself? You need to tame your ego. Practice deep breathing exercises to calm yourself, employing the meditation techniques we learned.

Exercise to relax your body and mind.

Take a break. Sometimes walking away from a tense situation is an effective way to calm yourself in a stressful situation. Putting yourself in a "time out" helps reduce stress. You will know when you are emotionally ready to revisit what was a tense situation.

Talk about your problems. Rather than leaning on yourself to cope with a mark of aging, it might prove fruitful to talk about your coping problems with a family member or a close friend.

Get enough sleep. Sleep deprivation makes us irritable and lowers our ability to cope—stress-free—with the marks of aging. Make sure you are getting at least 7 to 8 hours of sleep per night.

Decision-Making

The ability to make effective, well-thought-out decisions is key when coping with physical and mental decline as you age.

Decision-making consists of five steps:

➤ Identify your goal
➤ Gather information for weighing your options
➤ Consider the consequences
➤ Make your decision
➤ Evaluate your decision

Problem solving, an important part of decision-making, is the ability to find solutions to problems in situations where emotions are involved. Problem solving includes the ability to understand the impact that emotions can have on decision-making. (All our decisions are influenced by emotions to some degree.)

If you are feeling sad, you might be more willing to settle for things that aren't in your favor. Emotions can affect not just the nature of the decision, but the speed at which you make it. Anger can lead to impatience and rash decision-making. If you are afraid, your decisions may be clouded by uncertainty and caution, and it might take you longer to choose.

Hearing impairment is a great example of the role emotions play in decision-making. So many seniors delay wearing hearing aids due to embarrassment. Your ego is embarrassed, not you. Identify your goal: I want to hear! Gather information for weighing your options: Get a hearing test and compare the effectiveness and pricing of hearing aids. Consider the consequences: A hearing aid will improve quality of life. Make your decision: Acquire a hearing aid. Evaluate your decision: Quality of life improved.

The key is to remain objective in the decision-making process by seeing things as they really are. This capacity involves recognizing when emotions or personal bias can cause one to be less objective. To be an effective decision-maker, you must also resist or delay impulses or temptations to act without consideration. Objective decision-making is the key to successful aging.

Here are some ways to improve decision-making:

Exercise gets you in a more positive frame of mind with which to make decisions.

Social interaction. A healthy social life generates a positive framework for decision-making.

Take a big picture perspective. See the big picture when making an important decision. This is partially accomplished by writing down the benefits and costs of a situation.

Simplify the decision-making process. Simplify your decision by narrowing your options. Make the decision-making process as simple as possible.

Focus on what matters. Prioritize throughout the decision-making process. Don't sweat the small stuff—focus on what is truly important in your decision.

Self-Expression

Generally speaking, self-expression is the expression of one's feelings, thoughts, or ideas. Emotional expression is openly expressing one's feelings verbally and nonverbally.

For seniors aging, self-expression is the expression of one's own personality, an assertion of one's individual traits. Maintaining a high level of self-expression is crucial for seniors aging, since many seniors have difficulty maintaining their self-esteem and self-worth.

It is important for an older person to maintain some degree of independence and be self-directed and free from emotional dependence on others. How seniors share and express themselves to others forms the basis of their personality and sets the tone for how they live in their twilight years.

The journey of self-discovery is the most important journey we can take, especially as we are transitioning in our senior years. We don't want to lose our personality and the things that make us who we are as we age.

Here are some ways to improve self-expression:

Mental stimulation. Keep your mind alert by playing cards, puzzles, brain teasers, etc.

Read regularly.

Arts and crafts. Self-expression can be improved through an artistic activity such as arts and crafts.

Interpersonal

Interpersonal skills are what you use to interact with people. They help you develop and maintain mutually satisfying relationships that are characterized by trust and compassion.

Possessing interpersonal skills is crucial in a team-oriented work environment. However, as we learned in chapter 2: We Are in This Together, interpersonal skills are crucial for senior citizens seeking social support as they age in life. Social support matters when seniors are confronted with health issues because family and friends can help you manage the suffering and lift your spirit. We are all in this life together.

Interpersonal skills also include showing empathy—recognizing, understanding, and appreciating how other people feel—toward others. Empathy involves being able to articulate your understanding of another's perspective and behave in a manner that respect others' feelings.

Seniors who do well with aging tend to be social. They are just as open to hearing bad news as good news and they are experts at supporting themselves and others.

Seniors who possess good social skills are also good at managing change and resolving conflicts. They are excited about facing new challenges in aging. They are rarely satisfied with leaving things as they are, but they don't sit back and make others do the work.

There are many ways to maintain an active social life, including:

➤ Maintain close relations with family and friends
➤ Church and other support organizations
➤ Local community groups
➤ Stay active. Tennis, pickleball, golf, card games, etc.

Here are some ways we can build our social skills:

Self-confidence. If you are confident in yourself, you will have the right temperament to socialize with others.

Listening. Being a good listener will win you many friends.

Collaboration. The ability to work with other people is crucial to building and maintaining friendships.

Showing appreciation. Appreciating your family and friends ensures an active social life.

Positive attitude. Everyone wants to be around positive people.

CHAPTER THIRTEEN

Reclaim Your Life

I t's time to reclaim your life. In the previous chapters, you've learned all about the inevitable inconveniences of aging and the stages of transition. And you've seen how you can lean on your spirit and social network, and practice various methods of mindfulness and positivity so that you can avoid (or get out of) God's Waiting Room and age successfully in the Positive Aging Room.

So far, we've discussed a lot of spiritual and psychological steps you can take to reclaim your joy in living. In this chapter, I want to give you a few more practical steps that can help you reclaim your life—no matter what physical limitations you face.

MY JOURNEY

Reclaiming my life was my battle cry after cancer surgery. I had to deal with depression, anxiety, acid reflux, bile, stomach and intestines complications, and living on a feeding tube.

In addition to coping with these post-surgery complications and issues, I wanted to control my destiny and stop wallowing in self-pity. I found some activities to engage in that sent me on a new, satisfying journey in life. I've been through too much in my battle against cancer to lose control over my life now.

Positive Aging Activities

Positive aging activities are activities that help us maintain a happy and healthy lifestyle and make us feel good about ourselves as we inevitably experience physical and mental decline. With the right attitude and the right activities, we can avoid living in God's Waiting Room and enjoy and savor our remaining years on Earth.

Here are some practical activities you can engage in as you age. Some of these activities are designed to get you involved in a social network, while others are designed to lift your spirit while creating meaning and exhilaration in your life.

Challenge yourself: Celebrate your advancing years and commit to a new life. The inconveniences that come your way should not be an obstacle to participation. Whether you are in a wheelchair, undergoing cancer treatment, experiencing hearing loss, or enduring painful arthritis, these activities are designed to raise your spirit so you can battle your struggles with aging.

Our true regrets are those that stem from lack of effort. I've listed eight task areas that offer a host of activities that will help reclaim your life. Don't expect to do everything on the list; that would be unreasonable. These activities are also not for everyone. What works for me may not work for you, and I am currently limited in participating in some of the activities presented below due to the physical constraints from post-surgery complications. For the most part, a majority of the activities should be effective for everyone.

- ➤ Discover and Learn
- ➤ Fill a Hope Bucket
- ➤ Do Happy Things
- ➤ Seize Change
- ➤ Make a Difference
- ➤ Write a Bio Legacy
- ➤ Get to Know People
- ➤ Sounding Off

Discover and Learn

I've always been fascinated with the mysteries of life and the universe; it gets my adrenaline flowing. All truths exist in the universe; we just have to remove the cover to see them. The Earth has always orbited around the sun—we just needed Galileo Galilei's observations using a telescope to uncover this truth in the 1600s. There are many discovery activities to embrace. Hopefully, you will find some of the topics I'm learning about as exhilarating as I do.

History—Google different topics in history (e.g., the Roman Empire, the American Revolution)

Art museum—show and tell

Discovery Channel topics

Science/physics—great discoveries (e.g., Einstein's Theory of Relativity, string theory, black holes)

Fill a Hope Bucket

I placed this task second because hope brings new meaning to our lives. Hope helps you dream again, and there is no shortage of hopes or dreams for people over 50. So, go ahead and have a dream!

Start by creating a hope bucket list, which is a great way to add excitement into your life. You are not too old to do extraordinary—and sometimes stupid—things. Some ideas to consider adding to your hope bucket list include riding in a hot air balloon; getting a tattoo; riding an elephant; taking a trip to Africa; or rock climbing. I'm sure there are many items you would like to add to a hope bucket. Go ahead and create that list, start doing the things you hope to do, and fill that hope bucket so much that it overflows.

By the way, you may need a "dream team" made up of people who will help you and participate in filling your hope bucket. So, do a bit of planning for the things on your hope list you can't accomplish by yourself.

Do Happy Things

Many of us already do this task with enthusiasm every day. Call it a happiness project. Be happy *now*. Do happy things and prioritize happiness in your life. Entertain your friends. Favor activities with a goal, like cooking, reading, or crafts. If you are going to make friends, your objective is to discuss, discover, educate, and create happy moments with them. Learn something new about friends you've known for years. Laugh and find humor every day.

Seize Change

We live in a world of constant change and many of us in the over-50 crowd do not accept change easily, which puts us at a disadvantage as we grow older. If we do not keep pace with societal changes, we run the risk of becoming disenfranchised from society. The most visible example of the positive impact of embracing change is the iPhone. Ask any person over 50 how exhilarating it was when they first tried the iPhone. Changing with change helps keep you and your spirit alive.

Here are some suggestions for seizing change:

Show and tell with technology. Monitor changes in technology in different fields like science (space exploration), medicine (cyborgs), smartphones, computers, or whatever field interests you.

Follow the political scene in America. Following politics will be frustrating but also stimulating, and you will feel like part of the nation.

Experience virtual reality. If you don't have the money or time to travel long distances, climb on board the virtual reality train. Virtual reality is gaining in popularity. For starters, you can Google trips to India, China, and other exciting locations and watch videos. Soon you will be able to try virtual reality glasses where you feel like you've traveled to distant lands without ever leaving your home.

Make a Difference

People feel better about themselves when they meaningfully help other people or improve someone else's situations. The key is to make sure your spirit, and not your ego, is what's managing your make-a-difference activities. The ego may get you involved in these activities for the wrong reasons (attention or desire to be admired). In contrast, your spirit's intentions are sincerity and compassion. Participating in meaningful activities is, in effect, exercising your spirit. List a number of activities and ways to make a difference in the world, such as helping someone achieve their goals, serving your community, and donating your time to a charitable organization.

You don't have to find the cure for cancer or be the President of the United States. Serve on an advisory board or do service for your community. Outstanding public service takes many forms. Go to inner cities to build homes for the poor with Habitat for Humanity. Wherever your interests lie, you will find ways to help other people and at the same time help your country. Look in your newspaper for volunteer opportunities. Contact your local volunteer agency. See a need and fill it.

My make-a-difference activity was to create the nonprofit organization United We Age. At present, this organization consumes most of my time and fills me with hope and meaning.

Write a Bio Legacy

Everyone has a story, especially older people, because they have lived longer lives. Writing or reminiscing about your life history improves self-esteem and lessens stress and depression. It is a powerful activity for seniors needing a lift in life. If you don't like to write, you can produce your own video or audio bio legacy.

Many senior citizens seek meaning in the final phase of life. Telling your life story and sharing it with family and friends is a formal acknowledgment that your life is meaningful.

Google "bio legacy templates" and you will find templates outlining the categories that you may want to consider as you tell your life's story, such as family history, the middle years, retirement years, and reflections on your life. A bio legacy template that I recommend is presented in chapter 14, A Lifestyle Plan for Positive Aging.

Get to Know People

Put yourself in a position to meet people. You don't need to have an outgoing personality to do this. Think of it as a form of social discovery.

Don't take friends for granted. Friends are so valuable, yet we tend to forget their value because we're so wrapped up in our everyday world. Maybe you can create a group of your friends to socialize with on a regular basis. I'm a shy person and have avoided meeting new people in the past, but I've realized that when I meet people, I usually enjoy the experience. It's easy to avoid making friends in our senior years, an unfortunate consequence of living in a rut. This is something you need to correct if you are in this situation.

Sounding Off

My wife recently had to get an abscess drained. It is an incision and drainage procedure that is difficult to watch. The doctor locates the most protruding and bulging part of the abscess, pierces it with a scalpel, and drains the pus out. This is usually followed by some blood. This might be a crude analogy, but cancer patients experiencing intense chemotherapy and radiation treatment become emotional abscesses—at least I did. Life is so uncertain for most cancer patients that there were times when I just had to drain the emotional pus and vent about life. When I did, it made me feel better.

Vent about what you think is right about life and what you think is wrong. Vent about annoying people and vent about pleasant things. Venting does not have to be negative. You may have positive vents or negative vents; it depends on the subject matter. There is a wide range of topics that you could sound off on. Here are a few from my list:

- ➤ Politics: liberal views versus conservative views
- ➤ Racial tensions in America
- ➤ Religion
- ➤ ISIS/North Korea
- ➤ Kardashian craze
- ➤ Societal priorities (i.e., rewarding professional athletes/celebrities versus teachers/scientists)

A Journey for the Ages

I believe there are three guiding principles for positive aging:

- ➤ Aging is beautiful
- ➤ We are in this together—social support is necessary for maintaining quality of life
- ➤ A healthy spirit is your best friend

At some point in our lives, everyone will experience physical and mental decline (e.g., diabetes, dementia, Parkinson's, cancer, heart disease, hearing loss, mobility loss). Ancient Buddhism sought to address the issue of suffering 2,600 years ago. The afflictions from aging affect every family—no family escapes.

Although Buddhism (via its Four Noble Truths and Five Precepts) addresses how to deal with aging and suffering, it lacks practical solutions that we can apply in our daily lives as we experience the marks of aging. That's why I have filled this book with building blocks and practical actions—positive aging activities presented in this chapter—that you can take. I hope it helps you enjoy your journey for the ages.

MY JOURNEY

Positive aging saved my life. I am alive and stronger today because of positive aging. When I was diagnosed with stage 3 esophageal cancer, I was unprepared for battle. I had no knowledge or tools to effectively fight against a life-threatening disease. How do you prepare for chemotherapy and radiation treatment? How do you prepare for the aftermath of seven-hour esophagus and stomach surgery?

I hit bottom physically and emotionally. I experienced depression and a heightened anxiety and was close to taking permanent residence in God's Waiting Room. My stomach became inoperable; I was living on a feeding tube for over a year. My muscles atrophied; I lost twenty-five pounds and became an emaciated, broken man. Life was taken from me. Hovering over me like a dark cloud was the prospect that my cancer could return with a vengeance and eventually take my life. The curtains on my finality had been drawn wide open.

It was a long road to recovery, and it began with social support. My family and friends came to my rescue. It wasn't just the physical help of chores and hugs that helped me. It was their unqualified love that reenergized me, particularly my spirit.

Once my spirit awoke, I committed to helping myself. I learned to cope with aging and suffering by taking bits and pieces from Buddhism, New Age beliefs, positivity, mindfulness—the primary ingredients for positive aging. I also got involved in some activities presented in this chapter that helped my recovery enormously. I became inspired to live a full life and I had the knowledge and tools to make it happen.

My journey changed my life forever. Positive aging means having the right attitude about growing old. It is about maintaining a healthy lifestyle and staying engaged fully in life. My perspective about life has shifted. This is now for me a time for reflection and a time to give back to the community. It is also a time for relaxation and freedom. My children are grown, and I am free to travel or participate in my favorite activities. Maintain a positive attitude about life even as you experience physical and mental decline, so you don't lose control over your own life.

Our common goal is to live a more joyful life in our senior years. The secret is knowing that the marks of aging are inconveniences. I've come to the realization that a life of inconvenience is the new normal.

CHAPTER FOURTEEN

A Lifestyle Plan for Positive Aging

As we embark upon our final journey in life, we all desire to age gracefully, with dignity. Numerous practices and activities have been presented throughout this book to help you do just that. But you may be wondering where to start.

So, in this chapter, I present a number of lifestyle plans for positive aging. They are designed to get out ahead of the aging process and put us in the best possible position to effectively deal with the inconveniences of aging that will inevitably come our way.

A lifestyle plan promises to change your mindset and shift your perception about life into a new paradigm. The objective is to inspire and help you pursue a more joyful life as you age.

Let's face it, we all want to age successfully—but change is difficult, especially for older adults already set in their ways. I've found there are two commitments you need to make to create meaningful change. You must commit to making the change for yourself—it must come from inside you. But equally as important, change must be made for those you love the most.

This is particularly pertinent for older people who have families with children and grandchildren. You spent a great deal of energy and time loving and nurturing your extended family through the years, creating a magical bond between you and your family. It is in their best interest for you to age gracefully, living life to its fullest. And for those individuals that lack a large family, there are, hopefully, one or two family members (e.g., siblings) or close friends that fall into this category. It is fascinating how powerful our commitment is when we do things for people we love.

Going forward, we will no longer force change. We will promote acceptance as we head toward a fresh outlook and lifestyle in your life. So, hit the reset button. There are lifestyle changes you can make that will help you endure and thrive in your twilight years. Positive aging is a lifestyle and mindset designed for all of you who want to live life on your terms.

Why a Positive Aging Lifestyle Works

I have witnessed firsthand the challenges senior citizens face when experiencing physical and mental decline. Having volunteered for Meals on Wheels and for my own United We Age organization, I've seen my share of seniors residing in God's Waiting Room, the Practical Aging Room, and the Positive Aging Room. Additionally, I've spent a great deal of time visiting seniors living alone in their homes/apartments, as well as seniors residing in independent living, assisted living, and long-term care facilities. My experiences have helped me a great deal in identifying which lifestyles and behaviors are associated with the different aging rooms.

More important, my personal battle with stage 3 esophageal cancer has given me firsthand experience in facing and coping with many of the marks of aging. I learned a great deal from my journey and identified the building blocks of a positive aging mindset that helped me successfully cope with some of the most serious inconveniences (marks) of aging.

One final note: Some of you might approach the practice of positive aging with a skeptical eye. You might believe that you are able to cope quite effectively with, for example, hearing impairment. You are quite capable of purchasing a hearing aid to rectify the problem. But the overriding purpose of positive aging is to create a positive mindset and lifestyle so that when a mark of aging comes your way that you would have had difficulty coping with—for example, cancer—you are now well equipped to effectively manage the situation.

Introducing a Lifestyle Plan into Your Life

Practicing positive aging can begin at any age. The earlier in life that we integrate lifestyle changes consistent with positive aging, the greater likelihood of living a more joyful life. Although it is highly recommended for people over 50 to bring positive aging into their lives, any adult—whether 20, 30, 40 years old—would markedly improve the quality of their lives with a positive aging lifestyle and mindset.

So, let's introduce a lifestyle plan into your life. I have several plans to present, depending on a variety of factors. Selecting the right lifestyle plan depends on your current physical condition and mental state of mind. Are you anxious about growing old? Are you depressed about the prospects of finality? Do you lean heavily on religion? Are you in the early, middle, or late stages of aging? And, of course, do you currently reside in the Positive Aging Room or the Practical Aging Room or in God's Waiting Room?

No matter where you are in your life, I've found that strengthening your spirit as you experience physical and mental decline is critical to successful aging. So many people today are missing this. They do not acknowledge the importance and role that their spirits play in their lives. Hence, these lifestyle plans are designed to place a great emphasis on strengthening your spirit.

Select a plan and choose the practices and activities that satisfy your needs and physical and mental condition. These plans are presented to provide some structure in your life as you cope with the inconveniences of aging. Pick the plan that seems most appealing to you and follow it for a few weeks. Then assess your progress and determine if its working for you.

We begin with a Lifestyle Modifications Plan. At a minimum, everyone needs to integrate lifestyle modifications into their lives. This will create a positive mindset. Consider these modifications as creating the most basic lifestyle plan for positive aging.

The remaining lifestyle plans offered are plans targeted for helping you cope with the different categories of the marks of aging. We offer plans for individuals facing changes in:

> ➤ Physical appearance
> ➤ Bodily functions
> ➤ Mental health
> ➤ Disease/Illness

These targeted plans feature habits that will make a big difference and a number of activities/practices that promise to help you better cope with the inconveniences of aging. Many of the lifestyle changes presented work for me, and, hopefully, they will work for you. They are also constructed to be practical and easily implemented. Of course, you may customize these plans by replacing or adding other practices/ activities that meet your needs.

The Lifestyle Modification Plan

I offer lifestyle modifications for you to integrate into your everyday life. Adopt a lifestyle with these modifications and you will be endowed with a positive mindset, possessing the mental and emotional wherewithal to effectively cope with most inconveniences of aging that come your way.

Are you ready to commit to making positive changes to your current lifestyle? If so, here are ten lifestyle modifications that promise to set you up for success. I tried to make them as general as possible to make it easier and less confining for you to adopt these modifications in your everyday life.

Become More Spiritual

It is critical that you believe you are more than your physical body. Your spirit is unaffected by time and aging. You need to spend more time on your spiritual side. You need to strengthen your inner spirit as your physical body declines. Seek out moments that allow your spirit to reveal itself. Select one or more of the following ways to tap into and strengthen your spirit.

Meditation. Sit in a comfortable position and focus on clearing your mind for just a few minutes in the morning and evening. Doing this daily will strengthen your spiritual well-being.

Seek peaceful moments. At least once per day, put yourself in a place where you are away from all distractions: a peaceful place for you to ponder and summon your spirit.

Pray. Prayer is a profound way to tap into your spirit and communicate with what some believe to be godlike powers or a higher self.

Practice yoga, tai chi, qigong. Sometimes it is necessary to prepare your body for spiritual meditation. These three practices make it easier for you to process spiritual energy.

Stimulate your mind. Your mind is the gateway to your spirit, so stimulating it is essential for achieving your spiritual journey. Here are some ways to stimulate your mind that I believe are practical for aging individuals to implement: drawing/art, music, writing, mind games, and reading.

Stay Social

It is important to remain socially engaged for two reasons: Social support improves quality of life, and social interaction is a necessary component of your overall well-being. Select one or more activities to build a social support network as well as become socially active: family and friends, 55 + community, cards, travel group, church, other support organizations, community involvement.

Let Meditation into Your Life

Meditation is an effective way to tap into your spirit. It is an experience that clears your mind and brings you into focus with your spiritual side. Practice what I call simple meditation, to tap into and strengthen your spirit. Here is how to accomplish this:

> ➢ Take 2 to 5 minutes every morning and evening to meditate.
> ➢ Sit or lie comfortably and close your eyes.
> ➢ Breathe naturally and be aware of your breathing with each inhalation and exhalation.
> ➢ Optional: Repeat a mantra to yourself: Say "Ohm" or "I'm" repeatedly until you are in a slight peaceful awareness state.
> ➢ The morning meditation awakens your spirit to deal with your aging issues throughout the day. The evening meditation helps cleanse your ego's negative thoughts that have built up throughout the day.

Commit to Eating Healthier

Focusing on changing nutritional needs is a crucial step in managing individual health as we age. We recommend that you follow a healthier diet that includes some of the following foods: beans, green peas, grain products, cereal, oranges, limes, lemons, sweet peppers, strawberries, tomatoes, leafy greens, almonds, avocado, fish, spinach, and coffee. And take vitamin supplements for brain health: vitamins E, B6, B12, C, D, and omega-3 fatty acids.

Simplify Your Life

Learning ways to simplify your life is a must for individuals facing physical and mental decline. Simplifying your life for older persons reduces stress, anxiety, and depression. Here are some ways to simplify your life: less multitasking, organize the household, eliminate clutter, and downsize your living space.

Reduce Stress

A few minutes of practice per day can help reduce stress and anxiety. Here are some ways: meditate, stay calm, simplify your life, exercise, take a break, and get enough sleep

Stay in the Present Moment

Aging generally promises a simpler life that creates an opportunity to live in the present. Practice living in the present and you will minimize thoughts about your younger self, as well as reduce fears about the future. Here are some ways that people today live in the present: meditate, practice tai chi or qigong, block out past thoughts and worries about the future.

Stay Positive

Positivity is a powerful force to help you age successfully. For positivity to be effective, you need to make it a habit. This is accomplished over time by implementing daily positive practices in your daily life. Here are some habits you can integrate: repeat affirmations, lean on religion/supernatural (e.g., the Law of Attraction), focus on something positive, keep a gratitude journal, and calm your body.

Stay Healthy

A successful path toward positive aging includes addressing the health of your body and your emotions. You must practice healthy habits and maintain healthy nutrition to meet the needs of an aging physical body. Here are some of the best ways to keep your body as healthy as possible: simplify life, get enough sleep, keep structure in your life, practice proper posture, limit sitting, and follow a healthy nutrition plan (see Commit to Eating Healthier, above). And of course, exercise. For those of you in relatively good physical shape, weight lifting and treadmill jogging are effective ways to stay physically fit. For the rest of us, walking by counting steps keeps our physical bodies active and fit. According to the experts, you must walk at a minimum 5,000 steps per day to be labeled low active. An active senior walks 7,500 to 10,000 steps per day. Anything greater than 10,000 steps is a highly active workout for seniors.

Stay Balanced

People aging who lead well-balanced lives are at peace with themselves, while people who can't seem to find balance lead lives of disarray filled with stress, anxiety, and sometimes depression. The challenge is that we become increasingly out of balance as we age. Here are some ways to re-balance the composition of your life portfolio to better fit the new reality of life as an older person.

Expectations: Lower your expectations about how you expect your particular mark of aging (e.g., Parkinson's disease) to affect your quality of life in the future, or even eliminate expectations and create possibilities instead. For example, if you contract Parkinson's disease, lower your expectations about leading a normal physical life as you were accustomed to pre-Parkinson's and create a set of possibilities about what is possible for you to do going forward. You may no longer be able to participate in physical sports. Possibilities could include card games, chess, puzzles, and so on.

Lifestyle: You need to adjust your lifestyle. For example, if you experience Parkinson's disease or cerebral palsy, you may be confined to a wheelchair; you must accept this new way of life.

Social interaction: Are you participating in group activities? Do you attend church or other support organizations? Do you spend enough time with friends and family? You need to maintain an acceptable level of social interaction when stricken with a serious disease/illness; social support is critical.

Priorities: Prioritize your life in the following categories: goals in life, social interaction, your well-being, and happiness. Obviously, your priorities are turned upside down when faced with serious disease. (See the Life Balancing Audit later in this chapter.)

Lifestyle Plan for Physical Appearance

Coping with changes in physical appearance is primarily about your ego. To disarm the ego, you must summon and strengthen your spirit. Follow the lifestyle plan below and you will soon appreciate that you are more than your physical body.

Situation:

➢ You are likely experiencing difficulty coping with one or more of the following: wrinkles, age spots, turkey neck, graying or thinning hair, shrinkage, drooping nose/ears.

Goals:

➢ Push your ego aside and accept changes in physical appearance
➢ Become proud of your changing physical appearance

Action Items:
Tame ego
➢ Exercise 1
▪ Face your ego's negativity about aging head-on.
▪ Look in the mirror and notice everything old about you.
▪ Focus on your face and arms.

- Seek out wrinkles, skin blemishes, age spots, hair loss, and other marks.
- Tell your ego that you are proud of your marks of aging.
➢ Exercise II
  - Your ego loves company.
  - Identify famous people (e.g., entertainers, musicians, government leaders) who are aging.
  - Find common marks of aging that you have with them. It could be as simple as wrinkles or loss of hair.
  - Identifying with famous people helps your ego rationalize your struggles with changes in physical appearance.

Practice simple meditation to strengthen your spirit

➢ Take 2 to 5 minutes every morning and evening to meditate.
➢ Sit or lie comfortably and close your eyes.
➢ Breathe naturally and be aware of your breathing with each inhalation and exhalation.
➢ Repeat a mantra to yourself: Say "Ohm" or "I'm" repeatedly until you are in a slight peaceful awareness state.
➢ The morning meditation awakens your spirit to deal with your aging issues throughout the day. The evening meditation helps cleanse your ego's negative thoughts that have built up throughout the day.

Music
➢ Listen to music every day for 15 to 30 minutes or more.
➢ It can be jazz, classical, or even rock and roll or hip-hop, depending on your taste.
➢ Listening to music takes you into a slight meditative state, tapping into your inner spirit.

Acceptance
➢ Accept the inevitable changes to your physical appearance by using affirmations to create a positive mindset. Repeat the following affirmations on a daily basis:
  ▪ I am more than my physical body
  ▪ I am OK and accept myself as I age

Attitude
➢ Positive aging is about attitude. And it is acceptable to use your ego to exhibit attitude to confront societal forever-young attitudes that, for example, tell us that wrinkles and age spots are ugly. Repeat the following affirmations:
  ▪ Older people belong
  ▪ I am proud of my physical appearance

Stay in the present moment
➢ It is important to live in the present when experiencing a change in physical appearance. Block out past thoughts about when you were wrinkle-free and had a younger person's body. Thinking about the past will only increase stress and frustration. If possible, practice one or more of the following:
  ▪ Tai chi
  ▪ Qigong
  ▪ Yoga

Follow a well-being routine
➢ Taking care of your physical body improves self-confidence, helping you cope with appearance changes.
➢ Follow a healthier diet and maintain proper levels of vitamins A, B, B12, C, D and E. Also make sure you are getting enough calcium, fiber, protein, potassium, magnesium, and zinc.
➢ Exercise regularly with a combination of light aerobics (e.g., walking 5,000 to 10,000 steps per day) and weight resistance training (light dumbbells).

Recommended Routine

Wake-up hour:	Meditate for 2 to 5 minutes
Before lunch:	Conduct ego exercises 1 and 2
After lunch/dinner:	Repeat acceptance and attitude affirmations
	Exercise with aerobics (walking) or weight resistance training for 30 minutes
	Listen to music of your choice for 15 to 30 minutes.
1 time per week:	Participate in yoga, tai chi, qigong, or focus on blocking out past thoughts
Sleep hour:	Meditate for 2 to 5 minutes
All day:	Maintain a healthy diet throughout the day and walk between 5,000 to 10,000 steps per day.

Lifestyle Plan for Bodily Functions

A decline in bodily functions requires proper perspective. When you are confronted with a decline in a bodily function such as hearing impairment, rather than dwell on your inability to hear well, focus your attention on the good things in your life. Your bodily functions are something people take for granted until they lose them. Declining bodily functions diminishes quality of life—if you let it.

Situation:

➢ You are likely experiencing difficulty coping with one or more of the following: digestion, arthritis, mobility, hearing, vision, sleeping, sex drive.

Goals:

➢ Overcome shame and embarrassment
➢ Lessen stress and anxiety
➢ Stay positive and in the present moment
➢ Improve quality of life

Action Items:

 Tame ego

  ➩ Exercise I

   ▪ Your ego loves company

   ▪ Identify famous people currently or in the past (e.g., entertainers, musicians, government leaders) who have physical handicaps

   ▪ Find common marks of aging that you have with them. It could be as simple as a hearing aid, or as serious as using a walker/wheelchair (e.g., President George H Bush, President Franklin D Roosevelt)

   ▪ Identifying with famous people helps your ego rationalize your struggles with a decline in bodily function.

Practice simple meditation to strengthen your spirit

➩ Take 2 to 5 minutes every morning and evening to meditate.

➩ Sit or lie comfortably and close your eyes.

➩ Breathe naturally and be aware of your breathing with each inhalation and exhalation.

➩ Optional: Repeat a mantra to yourself: Say "Ohm" or "I'm" repeatedly until you are in a slight peaceful awareness state.

➩ The morning meditation awakens your spirit to deal with your aging issues throughout the day. The evening meditation helps cleanse your ego's negative thoughts that have built up throughout the day.

Go to a contemplative place

➩ Put yourself in a place where you can contemplate life by yourself for at least 15 to 30 minutes a day.

➩ It can be in your bedroom or on your back porch, or take a stroll down your street or in the park.

➩ The objective is to capture some moments when you can find peace of mind in a spiritual sense.

Acceptance
➤ Accept the inevitable changes to your bodily functions by using affirmations to create a positive mindset. Once you accept a bodily handicap such as mobility loss and accept that you can only walk using a walker, you are set up for success. Repeat the following affirmations daily:
  ▪ There are no such things as physical problems, only opportunities to overcome
  ▪ I love the challenges that aging presents.

Adaptation
➤ You must adapt to your physical handicaps.
  ▪ Adopt a practical approach to aging. Repeat the affirmation below every day:
  • I am flexible and adapt to change quickly.

Appreciation
➤ Appreciate life as an older person as your bodily handicaps mount. Have gratitude for the simple pleasures in life. Gratitude focuses on what is plentiful in your life, rather than what is missing (e.g., no longer being able to play tennis due to mobility loss).
  ▪ Write a gratitude journal weekly. Use the sample gratitude journal presented in the Resources section at the end of this chapter.

Attitude
➤ You possess value even with your bodily handicaps.
➤ Repeat the affirmation below daily:
  ▪ I am proud of my bodily handicaps because I can still smell the roses.

Stay in the present moment
➤ It is important to live in the present when experiencing a decline in a bodily function like mobility loss. Block out past

thoughts about when you were able to walk without the use of a walker. Thinking about the past will only increase stress and frustration. If possible, practice one or more of the following:

- Tai chi
- Qigong
- Yoga

Re-balance your life
➢ Changes in your bodily functions will likely set your life off balance, resulting in increased stress and frustration. Do the following to have a more balanced life:

- Conduct a **Life Balancing Audit** (available in the Resource section below)
- **Expectations:** lower your expectations about how you expect your affected bodily function to perform in the future, or even eliminate expectations and create possibilities instead. For example, if you experience mobility loss, lower your expectations about ever playing tennis again and create a set of possibilities about physical sports. Possibilities could include golf, pickleball, and so on.
- **Lifestyle:** You need to adjust your lifestyle. Examples are plentiful: If you experience mobility loss, get used to using a walker or wheelchair; if you experience hearing loss, wear a hearing aid; if you experience digestive problems when eating certain foods like pizza, eat the right foods.
- **Social interaction:** Are your participating in group activities? Do you attend church or other support organizations? Do you spend enough time with friends and family? You need to maintain an acceptable level of social interaction.
- **Priorities:** Prioritize your life in the following categories: goals in life, social interaction, your well-being, and happiness.

Engage in a Positive Aging Activity
➢ Two activities may help distract you as well as help you cope better with decline in bodily functions. Select one or both.
- Discover and learn
  - Google different topics in history (e.g., the Roman Empire, the American Revolution).
  - Visit an art museum.
  - Watch the Discovery channel on cable television.
  - Research the great discoveries in science (e.g., Einstein's Theory of Relativity, black holes in space).
- Seize change
  - Keeping informed about new developments in technology, politics, etc. keeps our minds fresh and open, distracting us and helping us cope better with the bodily function declines that are occurring.
  - Monitor changes in science, space exploration, medicine, smartphones, computers.
  - Follow the political scene in America.
  - Experience virtual reality. If you don't have the financial wherewithal to travel, use a virtual reality device to virtually take trips around the globe. See the Resources section at the end of this chapter for a list of virtual reality devices.

Follow a well-being routine
➢ Taking care of your physical body improves self-confidence, helping you cope with appearance changes.
➢ Follow a healthier diet and maintain proper levels of vitamins A, B, B12, C, D and E. Also make sure you are getting enough calcium, fiber, protein, potassium, magnesium, and zinc.
➢ Exercise regularly with a combination of light aerobics (e.g., walking 5,000 to 10,000 steps per day) and weight resistance training (light dumbbells).

Recommended Routine

Wake-up hour:	Meditate for 2 to 5 minutes
Before lunch:	Ego exercise I
After lunch/dinner:	Repeat adaptation and attitude affirmations
	Meditate for 30 minutes to practice mindfulness
	Go to your contemplative place for 15 to 30 minutes
1 time per week:	Assess your balanced life categories: expectations, lifestyle, social interaction, and life's priorities
	Write in your gratitude journal
1 time per month:	Participate in an activity: seize-change activities or discover-and-learn activities
Sleep hour:	Meditate for 2 to 5 minutes
Daily:	Walk between 5,000 to 10,000 steps per day.

Lifestyle Plan for Mental Health

Managing mental health issues is difficult and takes a special set of coping skills. And for dementia (e.g., Alzheimer's), some practices and activities are effective in the early stages but will most likely be ineffective in the later stages.

Situation:

➤ You are likely experiencing difficulty coping with one or more of the following: depression, anxiety, memory loss, dementia.

Goals:

➤ Accept and adapt to your memory loss and dementia
➤ Manage and lessen anxiety and depression
➤ Keep life simple and organized
➤ Eliminate embarrassment and raise self-esteem

Action Items:

Practice simple meditation to strengthen you spirit

- ➢ Take 2 to 5 minutes every morning and evening to meditate.
- ➢ Sit or lie comfortably and close your eyes.
- ➢ Breathe naturally and be aware of your breathing with each inhalation and exhalation.
- ➢ Repeat a mantra to yourself: Say "Ohm" or "I'm" repeatedly until you are in a slight peaceful awareness state.
- ➢ The morning meditation awakens your spirit to deal with your aging issues throughout the day. The evening meditation helps cleanse your ego's negative thoughts that have built up throughout the day.

Acceptance

- ➢ Accept the inevitable changes to your mental health by using affirmations to create a positive mindset. Repeat the following affirmation daily:
  - ▪ I am great and accept myself as I age.
- ➢ Memory loss is a permanent part of your life now and you need to accept your condition. View memory loss and dementia in a positive and possibly humorous light rather than as negative events.

Lifestyle changes

- ➢ Organized people live less stressful lives than people who are disorganized, and this is especially true for people experiencing serious memory loss and early dementia.
  - ▪ Create and follow daily routines
  - ▪ Do less multitasking; live a simpler life

Follow a well-being routine for dementia

- ➢ Taking care of your physical body improves self-confidence, helping you cope with appearance changes.

➢ Follow a healthier diet that includes some of the following foods: beans, green peas, grain products, cereal, oranges, limes, lemons, sweet peppers, strawberries, tomatoes, leafy greens, almonds, avocado, fish, spinach, and coffee.

➢ Take vitamin supplements for brain health: vitamins E, B6, B12, C, D, and omega-3 fatty acids.

➢ Exercise regularly is good for brain health; walk between 5,000 to 10,000 steps per day.

➢ Rest when possible.

➢ Treat hearing loss promptly. Hearing loss is sometimes associated with dementia.

Mind stimulation activities—select one or more of the following:
➢ Drawing/art
➢ Music
➢ Writing
➢ Mind games (puzzles, chess, card games)
➢ Reading

Use a note/memory reminder calendar (read more about this calendar in the Resources section at the end of the chapter under the "Memory Loss/Dementia Aids" heading.

Use a medical pill weekly container for taking medication daily.

Age-related depression
➢ Depression can be triggered by a midlife crisis or upon retirement, or it could be triggered anytime a person realizes that his or her life has less meaning than it once had.

➢ If you are feeling sadness, hopelessness, and emptiness, or heightened anxiety and an indifference to making decisions, you need to see a medical professional.

➢ In addition to medical assistance from professionals, the following ways should help you avoid or minimize age-related depression:

- Socialize
- Maintain structure in your life
- Continue employment
- Get involved in community service
- Continue to learn

Recommended Routine

Wake-up hour:	Meditate for 2 to 5 minutes
Before lunch:	Write in your note reminder calendar what to do for the day/week
	Participate in one of the mind-stimulating activities (art, music, writing, mind games, reading)
	Take you meds from the med pill weekly container
After lunch/dinner:	Repeat all the affirmations for your mental health
1 time per week:	Review your daily routines and make changes if necessary
	For age-related depression, select a way to minimize depression (socialize, maintain structure in your life, continue employment, get involved in community service, continue to learn)
Sleep hour:	Meditate for 2 to 5 minutes
Daily:	Follow your well-being routine

Lifestyle Plan for Disease/Illness

Many of us eventually experience true suffering: disease or serious illness. These are the most difficult of the inconveniences of aging. In many cases, individuals stricken with serious disease experience a mix of shame, embarrassment, anxiety, and depression, not to mention fear of the unknown. Constructing an effective lifestyle plan for disease/illness is critical for you to live life to its fullest under such trying conditions.

Situation:

> You are likely experiencing difficulty coping with one or more of the following: cancer, heart disease, Parkinson's disease, multiple sclerosis, and equally debilitating conditions.

Goals:

> Maintain meaningfulness in your life
> Remember that you are more than your physical body
> Stay positive
> Live in the present, not the past or future
> Overcome embarrassment or depression

Action Items:

Tame ego

> Exercise I
  - Your ego loves company
  - Identify famous people (e.g., entertainers, musicians, government leaders) who have or experienced serious disease/illness (e.g., Michael J. Fox with Parkinson's disease).
  - Identifying with famous people helps your ego rationalize your struggles with aging.

Practice mindfulness (advanced meditation) to strengthen you spirit and live in the present moment. Take at least 30 minutes every morning and evening to meditate.

> Sit or lie comfortably and close your eyes.
> Breathe naturally and be aware of your breathing with each inhalation and exhalation.
> Repeat a mantra to yourself: Say "Ohm" or "I'm" repeatedly until you are in a slight peaceful, awareness state.

➤ The morning meditation awakens your spirit to deal with your aging issues throughout the day. The evening meditation helps cleanse your ego's negative thoughts that have built up throughout the day.

➤ This meditation helps you attain a mindfulness state, helping you live in the present moment as well as awakening your spirit.

Optional spiritual practices:

➤ Conduct an out-of-body experience using the Monroe Hemi Sync method

➤ Utilize crystals to tap into your spirit

- Acquire a crystal of your choice. Select from among the five crystals presented in this book: clear quartz, selenite, shungite, amethyst, citrine. (For descriptions, see chapter 3, The Power of Me: Inner Spirit.)

- For believers, you will connect with your crystal and feed off its emission of positive energy, lifting vibrations and moving you to a higher spiritual state.

- Put your crystal into practice by wearing it as jewelry, carrying it in your pocket, or placing it in your home.

➤ Lean on prayer

➤ Practice yoga

➤ Seek peaceful moments

- Put yourself in a place where you can contemplate life by yourself for at least 15 to 30 minutes.

- It can be in your bedroom or on your back porch, or take a stroll down your street or in a park.

- The objective is to capture some moments when you can find peace of mind.

➤ Practice tai chi or qigong

Acceptance

➤ Accept the inevitability of your disease/illness by using affirmations to create a positive mindset. Repeat the following affirmation daily:

- I am more than my physical body.

Music
- ➤ Listen to music every day for 15 to 30 minutes or more.
- ➤ It can be jazz, classical, or even rock and roll or hip-hop, depending on your taste.
- ➤ Listening to music takes you into a slight meditative state, tapping into your inner spirit.

Find meaning in life
- ➤ Engage in community service
- ➤ Volunteer for a charitable organization
- ➤ Be active in church and other support organizations
- ➤ Be a big brother/sister for at-risk teenagers

Leave a legacy
- ➤ Leave a social legacy (e.g., becoming president of a local club, volunteering for a local charitable organization).
- ➤ Leave of family legacy (e.g., leaving a family business to your children)

Lean on religious or supernatural practices
- ➤ Traditional religion: Christianity, Judaism, Islam
- ➤ Eastern religious beliefs (e.g., Buddhism; Hinduism)
- ➤ New Age beliefs (e.g., the Law of Attraction)

Re-balance your life
- ➤ A serious disease/illness creates a major imbalance in your life, resulting in increased stress and frustration. Do the following to have a more balanced life:
  - ▪ Conduct a **Life Balancing Audit** (available in the Resource section below)
  - ▪ **Expectations:** Lower your expectations about how you expect your particular disease (e.g., cancer) to affect your quality of life in the future, or even eliminate expectations and create possibilities instead. For example, if you

contract Parkinson's disease, lower your expectations about leading a normal physical life that you were accustomed to pre-Parkinson's and create a set of possibilities about what is possible for you to do going forward. For example, you may no longer be able to participate in physical sports. Possibilities could include card games, chess, puzzles, and so on.

- **Lifestyle:** You need to adjust your lifestyle. Examples are plentiful: If you experience Parkinson's disease or cerebral palsy, you may be confined to a wheelchair; you must accept this new way of life.

- **Social interaction:** Are your participating in group activities? Do you attend church or other support organizations? Do you spend enough time with friends and family? You need to maintain an acceptable level of social interaction when stricken with a serious disease/illness; social support is critical.

- **Priorities:** Prioritize your life in the following categories: goals in life, social interaction, your well-being, and happiness. Obviously, your priorities are turned upside down when faced with serious disease.

Write a bio legacy
- ➢ Reminiscing about your life history improves self-esteem and lessens stress and depression. This is a powerful activity for helping individuals cope with changes in physical appearance. It is an effective distraction and confidence booster.
- ➢ Google "bio legacy template" and you will find templates outlining a bio legacy, or follow the bio legacy outline presented in the Resource section at the end of this chapter.

Follow a well-being routine
- ➢ Taking care of your physical body improves self-confidence, helping you cope with appearance changes.

➤ Follow a healthier diet and maintain proper levels of vitamins A, B, B12, C, D and E. Also make sure you are getting enough calcium, fiber, protein, potassium, magnesium, and zinc.

➤ Exercise regularly with a combination of light aerobics (e.g., walking 5,000 to 10,000 steps per day) and weight resistance training (light dumbbells).

Recommended Routine

Wake-up hour:	Meditate for 30 minutes
Before lunch:	Repeat affirmations for acceptance
After lunch/dinner:	Conduct ego exercise
1 time per week:	Monitor and review life balance (adjust expectations, lifestyle, social interaction, and priorities)

Work on your bio legacy

1 time per month: Select an optional spiritual practice (OBE; crystals; prayer; yoga; peaceful moments; tai chi/qigong)

Select a meaningful activity (community service; church; big brother/sister volunteer work)

Sleep hour:	Meditate for 30 minutes
Daily	Practice religious/supernatural/Eastern religious beliefs/New Age beliefs

Acquire crystals, or conduct out-of-body experiences, or lean on prayer, or practice yoga, or go to a contemplative place, or practice tai chi/qigong.

Follow a well-being routine

Final Thoughts

Hopefully, there is a lifestyle plan that meets your needs, taking you on a wondrous journey of aging. I urge everyone reading this book to take the plunge and commit to one or more of the positive aging lifestyle plans presented in this chapter.

At the very least, I implore you to give the lifestyle modifications plan your best effort. Incorporating these modifications into your everyday life will pay enormous dividends as you experience physical and mental decline.

None of us escapes the tight grasp of Father Time, and unfortunately for us, Father Time is undefeated. It is figuratively written in stone: All of us are destined to grow old and not be able to do the things we were able to do in our youthful years.

Here's my two cents: Go 10,000 feet in the air and look at the big picture of your life. Then select the lifestyle plan and the specific activities/practices that best meet your goals and objectives. Planning and organizing your time and tracking your progress are the keys to accomplishing your positive aging goals.

Resources for Positive Aging Lifestyle Plans

Practicing a positive aging lifestyle plan requires that you engage in a number of practices and activities every day, week, month, and year. Fortunately, there are resources available for you to facilitate the implementation of the plans. Presented below are resources for:

➢ Meditation
➢ Out-of-body experiences
➢ Virtual reality
➢ Gratitude journal
➢ Memory loss/dementia
➢ Bio legacy template
➢ Life Balancing Audit

Meditation (Apps)

The following apps offer a variety of meditation exercises including mindfulness, spiritual awakening, stress, sleep, positivity, anxiety, happiness, and wellness

- ➢ Calm
- ➢ Simple Habit
- ➢ Waking Up
- ➢ UCLA Mindful
- ➢ Headspace
- ➢ hemi-sync.com

Out-of-Body Experiences

- ➢ Hemi Sync OBE: Guided meditation into out-of-body experiences and astral projection

Virtual Reality

- ➢ Oculus Go Standalone VR Headset
- ➢ HTC Vive Cosmos VR Headset
- ➢ Oculus Quest All-in-One VR Gaming Headset

Gratitude Journal (Apps)

- ➢ Grateful: A Gratitude Journal
- ➢ Gratitude Happiness Journal
- ➢ Happyfeed: Daily Gratitude Journal

Memory Loss/Dementia Aids

A number of traditional memory aids may help a person with memory problems, such as writing things in a diary or calendar, or using an automatic calendar clock.

Elevate Brain Training app: Play games to improve focus, memory, speaking, mental math, and more.

Medication Reminder Box: A great tool for any senior. It features different compartments for each day and for all the different pills that need to be taken that day.

Smartphone alarms: Seniors with memory issues/dementia can benefit from smartphones and use daily alarms as a reminder for what they need to do that day.

Portable notepads: Seniors with memory problems/dementia can use a notepad to write themselves notes on what they need to do, etc.

Calendar: Place a calendar where a senior with dementia can see it every day. The calendar should include doctor appointments, social engagements, and so on.

Memory Reminder Apps:
- ➢ To Do Reminder with Alarm
- ➢ Reminder with Voice Reminders
- ➢ TickTick
- ➢ Remember the Milk
- ➢ Todoist
- ➢ Google Keep
- ➢ Evernote

Bio Legacy Template

Family History
- ➢ When and where were you born?
- ➢ Where is your family from/what is your heritage?
- ➢ Other…

Early Years–Childhood
- ➢ What was your first memory as a child?
- ➢ What do you recall of your early education?
- ➢ What did your parents do for a living?
- ➢ Other…

The Teenage Years
> ➤ Memories of school
> ➤ What were your favorite pastimes as a teenager?
> ➤ Who were your best friends?
> ➤ Other...

The Middle Years
> ➤ Did you go to college or get a job?
> ➤ When did you get married?
> ➤ Who were your best friends?
> ➤ Talk about your children, if you had any
> ➤ Talk about your work. What type of job did you have?
> ➤ Any interesting stories about your job?
> ➤ Other...

Retirement Years
> ➤ When and why did you decide to retire?
> ➤ What were your retirement plans; did you achieve them?
> ➤ Travel; favorite pastimes

Reflections on Your Life
> ➤ If you could, would you do some things differently?
> ➤ Who was the love of your life?
> ➤ What is your greatest achievement/failure?
> ➤ Other. . .

Life Balancing Audit

(Sample)

To conduct a personal audit of your life, it might be useful to complete the Life Balancing Audit chart below. Rank each life category using the levels High, Good, Fair, and Poor. Please be as objective about your life as you can. After assessing your personal life audit, identify the re-balancing steps necessary to bring better equilibrium to your life.

	Level
Balance Indicator	
➢ Stress level:	High
➢ Anxiety level:	High
➢ Depression:	Low
Expectations	High
Lifestyle	
➢ Diet	Poor
➢ Choices	Good
➢ Exercise	Poor
➢ Activities	Fair
➢ Organization	Poor
Social Interaction	
➢ Family/friends	Good
➢ Group activities	Good
➢ Church/orgs	Fair
Priorities	
➢ Well-being	Poor
➢ Social interaction	Good
➢ Goals	Fair
➢ Happiness	Poor

Re-balancing Steps
- ➢ Need to lower expectations in my life
- ➢ Reduce anxiety/stress
  - ▪ Exercise regularly
  - ▪ Improve organization/simplify my life
- ➢ Place greater emphasis on well-being
  - ▪ Improve diet
  - ▪ Exercise regularly
  - ▪ Do happy things

CHAPTER FIFTEEN

Aging in America

The preceding chapters laid out a road map for individuals to practice positive aging. Hopefully, you discovered the power of positive aging, and you are well on your way to a more joyful life in your senior years.

This chapter is focused less on individuals and more on our society. We are all living in a society that demonstrates little value for aging or the elderly. Better understanding the society around us helps us cope better with the bewildering changes we are facing. And—hopefully—as more of us reject our society's forever-young attitude, we can help our society become a better place to grow old.

Not everyone is able to age successfully in America. As we learned thus far, if you are fortunate enough to have a family/friend support network, you are on your way toward positive aging. Positive aging works if we have social support to help raise our spirits. Unfortunately, there are too many people aging alone who have little or no social support. Without the help of others, their quality of life suffers. These older adults are unable to discover the power of positive aging. There is an "alone crisis" in America today. Furthermore, older people, whether alone or with family or friends, face ageism as well as forever-young attitudes, which negatively affect senior citizens' self-worth and behavior. These are the primary aging issues facing senior citizens today.

➢ The alone crisis
➢ Ageism
➢ Forever-young attitudes

The Alone Crisis

The alone crisis affects millions of older adults across the nation. Nobody should grow old alone; nobody should experience a life-threatening disease alone. Social support saved my life—it gave me confidence to battle cancer and lifted my spirit to regain my passion to live. Without social support, people aging alone are not likely to have the opportunities and the positive aging tools to live joyful lives.

Millions of senior citizens are residing in long-term care facilities or small, run-down apartments or homes. They have little or no social support and are financially challenged. In fact, according to Adopt a Senior, there are about 3 million older adults living in long-term care/nursing facilities and almost half of them do not have any family or friends visit them throughout the year.[40]

According to the 2018 Profile of Older Americans, almost 30 percent (14.3 million) of noninstitutionalized older people (65+) live alone in the United States today. Almost half of older women (44 percent) age 75+ live alone. For older people in 2017 (50.9 million), 13 percent reported income of less than $10,000. The median income for older people was reported at $24,224.[41]

Quality of life and even life expectancy suffer tremendously for older people and people stricken with life-threatening diseases who live alone and lack social support (i.e., a spouse, family member, or caring friend). In the case of a life-threatening disease like cancer, studies suggest that social support (particularly a spouse) matters more than chemotherapy.

According to most research studies (e.g., Macmillan Cancer Support Study), people who lack social support networks are three times more likely to struggle to follow their treatment plan than those who aren't lonely.[42]

For example, more than one in five cancer patients (22 percent) experience loneliness following diagnosis, and those who are lonely are nearly three times more likely to have issues with following their treatment plan than those who aren't lonely (31 percent vs. 11 percent).

Further, a New York University Lagone Medical Center study (2014) found that married people (a proxy for social support) had a 5 percent lower risk of cardiovascular disease compared to single people. The project is the largest study to ever look at the link between marriage and heart health. The study looked at 3.5 million American adults and found that married people have lower odds of cardiovascular disease than those who are single, divorced, or widowed.[43]

Even with outstanding local organizations there is not enough support for older or disabled people living alone. A social worker can only do so much. Further, our medical system caters to the very needy, so it might take care of you only if you are critically ill or provide financial support only if you are impoverished. Getting personal home care is expensive, ranging from $16 to $28 per hour (depending on location), which most people can't afford.[44] There is currently a shortage of home care workers, and it's going to get worse. According to the Institute of Medicine, by 2030, the United States will need 3.5 million more workers in home care and geriatric medicine than what is currently available, while the elderly population is expected to double by 2050.[45]

The alone crisis is only going to get worse because of changing family dynamics. According to a 2016 Study by the National Academy of Sciences, families have fewer children, older adults are more likely to have never married or to be divorced, and adult children often live far from their parents or may be caring for more than one adult or their own children.[46]

The private sector isn't a great option for many older adults. Demand for caregivers will exceed supply by more than 3 million in the next decade. More important, baby boomers, who are often today's caregivers, are going to need care and social support as they age into their golden years. For many, it is unclear who will provide care and social support.

The severity of the alone crisis is in the numbers: About 14 percent of frail older adults, 2 million people, are without children and the number is expected to double by 2040, according to the AARP Public Policy Institute.[47] There is no natural caregiver or social support for this population group.

The results of a decades-long study from the University College London on the impact of loneliness and isolation has shown that both loneliness and infrequent contact with friends and family can shorten a person's life.[48]

With the 65+ population in the United States poised to grow to over 70 million from 40 million over the next several decades—combined with life-threatening diseases (e.g., Alzheimer's, cancer) set to double in cases over the same period—the problem is only going to get worse. Who is going to care for single baby boomers as they face the inevitable decline of old age? If you show the way by helping an aging person in need, perhaps there will be someone to help you when you experience the marks of aging.

Ageism

A primary stumbling block to appropriate care and social support for the elderly is ageism, which is widespread in our society. Ageism is discrimination against older adults and has a severe effect on the self-esteem and well-being of our senior citizen population; it is particularly hard on older adults who lack social support (family/friends). Or more specifically, it is discrimination against persons of a certain age group—a tendency to regard older people as debilitated, unworthy of attention, or unsuitable for employment. Ageism refers to the negative attitudes, stereotypes, and behaviors directed toward older adults based solely on their perceived age.

Evidence of ageism can be observed especially in the workplace and health-care facilities. However, our focus is on how ageism affects an older person's ability to cope with aging.

According to a study by Becca Levy,[49] negative stereotyping is hurtful to older people and even shortens their lives. The study observed 660 people 50 years and older. Those with positive self-perceptions of aging lived 7.5 years longer than those with negative self-perceptions of aging. People's positive beliefs about and attitudes toward older adults appear to boost their mental health. Older adults exposed to positive stereotypes had significantly better memory and balance, whereas negative self-perceptions contributed to poorer memory and feelings of worthlessness.

Ageism or the stigma of aging is something all of us must fight through. Younger people stereotype older people, which makes it difficult for aging adults to stay positive about growing old.

Although there are exceptions to perceptions of older adults—like the "grandmother" subtype, who is viewed as kind, nurturing, and helpful; or the "elder statesmen" subtype, who is viewed as competent, intelligent, and wise—the bulk of aging senior citizens are viewed in a negative light.

As a population segment, senior citizens constitute a devalued group in society and culture, but there are remedies and interventions for improving these perceptions. Improving positive attitudes toward older adults will improve senior citizens' lives. According to Avshalom Caspi, children with daily contact with older adults at their preschool were found to hold positive attitudes toward older adults, whereas children without such contact held vague or indifferent attitudes.[50]

Similarly, the Dasgupta and Greenwald 2001 study found that young adult participants revealed less automatic age bias if they had recently been exposed to admired older adult exemplars (e.g., Mother Teresa) and disliked young exemplars (e.g., Tonya Harding), compared to recent exposure to disliked older adult exemplars and admired young exemplars. This research suggests that exposure to positive models of older people may reduce bias and stereotyping toward that group. To me, this suggests that a media campaign promoting positive senior citizen models is a step in the right direction in reversing negative stereotyping of the older adult population group.[51]

If there is one common thread across ageism studies over the past twenty years, it is that older adults with more positive self-perceptions and views of aging have better physical health and better survival rates than those with more negative self-perceptions and views. And according to a study by N. Krause in 1987, negative views about aging predict low self-esteem and high levels of depression among older adults.[52]

Forever-Young Attitudes

Fueling the problem of ageism is the media's portrayal of older adults. In many cases, we are brought to believe that older adults are dependent, helpless, unproductive, and ugly (due to wrinkling and graying). The value that the media and society place on youthfulness partially explains the growing antiaging industry with its antiaging creams and cosmetic surgery.

So, older adults face an external obstacle—forever-young attitudes—obfuscating their ability to cope effectively with the marks (inconveniences) of aging. As mentioned elsewhere, for many of us, aging is like swimming upstream against the current in today's forever-young society. People spend billions of dollars on antiaging creams and surgical procedures to eliminate the worn look of wrinkles rather than choosing to view wrinkled faces as reflections of life's experiences that took years to create.

It bears repeating that there is nothing inherently wrong with wanting to appear young if it makes you feel good, raises your confidence, and promotes a healthier lifestyle. The problem with the forever-young attitude is not individual attempts to maintain a youthful appearance but rather the societal messaging that staying young is superior to growing old.

Of course, older adults' perceptions of their future selves play a major role here as well. Too many older adults possess a diminished self-worth and engage in societal isolation or depression in today's forever-young society. The objective is to age with a positive attitude in a society that emits negative messaging toward older adults. This is a difficult task and one that has been the primary subject of this book. A more age-friendly society would create a culture of celebration and respect for older people across the nation, and we will all grow old gracefully with dignity. Winston Churchill once said, "Attitude is a small thing that makes a big difference." People may hear your words, but they feel your attitude.

The consequences of forever-young attitudes for the opportunities and life outcomes of older adults are real. Research reveals that forever-young societal attitudes negatively influence the life outcomes of older adults, directly as well as through life-expectancy effects and self-stereotyping. This exerts greater importance on utilizing the tools presented in this book to cope effectively with the inconveniences of aging.

Proposed Solutions

The solution, of course, is to eliminate forever-young attitudes and ageism in America, as well as provide greater social support to older adults living alone.

Ageism in America and forever-young attitudes are major stumbling blocks for the happiness of older adults. There have been some positive steps in changing societal attitudes, such as the portrayal of gray hair as powerful and beautiful in advertising. This has shifted the perception toward aging ever so slightly. But more fundamental changes in societal attitudes toward aging need to be made in order to cope with the vulnerabilities of an increasingly aging society.

Improve Social Support

We also need a call to action to help the millions of older people with little social support. A medical practitioner or social worker can only do so much. Often, after a cancer patient or an older person with quality of life issues visits a social worker or medical practitioner, they return home to a lonely void.

Aging people need a social network (family and friends), and if that doesn't exist, we need to build a social network for them. Educating younger generations about aging is a good start. The medical community needs to target the people who don't have support and seek help from local community services. It is difficult to be the doctor/nurse, caregiver, and advocate all at one time.

Imagine a movement where the younger generations are more aware and supportive of people aging. There are 75 million Millennials (born 1981 to 1997) in the United States and over 65 million Generation Xers (born 1965 to 1980). These generations of people could have a positive impact on the lives of older generations for years to come.

The medical community needs to be aware that patients who live alone are at risk for worse outcomes, and it should try to do things to make up for the relative lack of support.

We need to build local social networks across the nation to help people facing quality-of-life decline. Although many organizations offer social support through staff (e.g., case workers) and volunteers, too many people continue to age alone. Even people living in senior living facilities who are not physically alone may be emotionally alone. We need to offer companionship to people who are alone, and we need to advocate on their behalf.

Promote Active Aging

We need to create a culture that promotes active and healthy aging and influences older people's health and quality of life. And we need to create age-friendly communities and maximize awareness about aging and social participation.

We need to raise awareness by mobilizing people across generations to get involved in the aging process. All young people have parents and grandparents who experience the marks of aging: some-one in a senior living community, someone with cancer, someone with loss of mobility, someone with hearing loss, or someone who just died. We need to share stories so everyone can feel united and to create a comfort level that we are all in this together.

Educate Young People

We need to educate younger people, and older people, on how to deal with the marks of aging (suffering) and the final transition. We need to support research that demonstrates the positive correlation between positivity and success; social support and success; and social accep-tance and success. The two measures of success are improved quality of life and extended life expectancy.

We need to teach society that aging is a beautiful process, if we can emotionally manage physical and mental health decline. Transi-tioning to the other side, no matter what your religious or scientific beliefs, is a process of acceptance.

We need to change societal attitudes and images of aging and cancer/life-threatening disease victims. We need to change cultural practices regarding the marks of aging. We live in a forever-young society, even though we should be living in a forever-aging society. Why can't we have it both ways? Why can't we blend forever-young with forever-aging? Let's celebrate both together.

CHAPTER SIXTEEN

United We Age

I've founded a nonprofit organization called United We Age to create a more positive and supportive aging environment in America. It is my response to the issues raised in the previous chapter that are the primary societal hurdles facing senior citizens today: the alone crisis, ageism, and forever-young attitudes.

Here are some action steps that are included on the organization's agenda.

Create a Social Support Network

Urge people of all generations to join a "united we age" movement. This support network provides people living alone with companionship and guidance for improving quality of life and life expectancy as they experience the marks of aging or experience life-threatening diseases/conditions.

United We Age, UWA, will recruit and train younger population groups (e.g., Millennials and Generation Xers) as well as baby boomers to become part of a united movement so they better understand and participate in the aging process. We need to recruit volunteers from all population groups, so everyone in society is engaged with aging. The stigma of aging is eliminated when people work together to help everyone age with joy and dignity.

The goal is to create a network of nonprofessionals—regular people—to join a "friends for seniors" system for older people living alone or who lack any meaningful family/friend support. This system could be similar to today's Big Brothers and Big Sisters of America, whose volunteers serve as older siblings to at-risk teenagers. UWA volunteers are people who care about other people's quality of life. They will communicate with the case workers and other professional volunteers about an older person's situation. Volunteers effectively befriend an older person in need. They help seniors make better informed decisions about quality-of-life concerns. They may invite seniors home for a holiday like Thanksgiving or Christmas, look in on them, talk to a case worker, and make sure the seniors are getting the right medical and emotional attention, such as lifting their spirit.

Raise Awareness and Improve the Image

It's not senior citizens who are old; attitudes toward senior citizens are old. Changing this begins with changing the image of older people. In marketing terms, we need to change the brand. For the past century, senior citizens have been branded as old, frail, useless, and helpless, among other derogatory adjectives. Our goal is to brand older people as dynamic individuals who are full of life, passion, and pride.

There have been some positive steps in changing societal attitudes, such as the portrayal of gray hair as powerful and beautiful in advertising. This has shifted the perception toward aging ever so slightly. Fundamental changes in societal attitudes toward aging need to be made in order to cope with the vulnerabilities of an increasingly aging society.

It will take a concerted effort to shift people's views of an entire class of people. Media campaigns could include a combination of advertisements, op-eds, articles, and press releases using the full spectrum of media: television, radio, print, and social media.

A successful public relations campaign will replace a forever-young society with a society that honors and reveres its aging population.

This is a battle over lives, and it takes all of us working together to make it happen.

We should also highlight the potential commercial value of the senior population, which holds around $9 trillion in net assets. This staggering amount should capture the attention of business and government leaders.

Elevate National Senior Citizens Day. Ever since President Ronald Reagan on August 19, 1988, proclaimed August 21 as National Senior Citizens Day, the public has largely ignored the holiday. We need to raise awareness of this holiday by celebrating older Americans' contributions to their country and communities.

Endorsements from celebrities, business leaders, and government leaders will increase our movement's visibility and encourage millions of people to get involved.

Create and produce a documentary on aging in America exposing the harsh reality that too many older people and people with life-threatening disease live alone, in a forever-young society that doesn't respect or revere older people.

Research and Educate

Conduct surveys and research to support our proclamations about the negative effects of antiaging sentiment on senior citizen life. Support research that demonstrates the positive correlation between social support and quality of life/life expectancy.

Create a grassroots initiative designed to increase awareness of aging among all generations of people through social education. The aim is to raise awareness of underlying ageism in the community and how it contributes to a negative view of older people. Encourage younger generations to join support networks.

Develop education curriculum and programs to teach and train younger people and older people how to deal with and manage the marks of aging. We train people to be doctors, lawyers, and construction workers but we do not train people how to grow old.

Final Thoughts

My hope is to inspire Americans regardless of age to join a United We Age movement. Almost 40 million people are considered senior citizens (65+) in America today. With 76 million aging boomers, the senior citizen population is poised to represent almost 20 percent of the total population by 2030. Together we can make a difference in their lives.

Our culture needs to redefine successful aging. It is not simply a post-retirement life. It is not simply fulfilling a bucket list or participating in community activities, although those are steps in the right direction.

A pro-aging culture respects and celebrates the lives of its senior citizens and acknowledges the physical, mental, and emotional transitions that older people experience. These considerations are important in a society with a senior population that is projected to explode. After all, the fate of older people is a personal one, since we are all destined to become senior citizens.

In a youth-obsessed society, older people's social worth declines with age. Put yourself in an older person's shoes—experience some of the inconveniences of aging along with the anxiety and sometimes depression that comes with aging—and you will gain a better understanding of what it's like to grow older.

Older citizens are also at the mercy of an unresponsive legislative body, a younger generation that doesn't understand, appreciate, or value the contributions of those who came before them, and a medical system that's under financial stress through no fault of its own.

As stated elsewhere, there are many organizations (such as AARP, Meals on Wheels, Community Care Program, Caregiver Action

Network, to name a few) helping older people live better lives every day, offering health care, home care, and other support services, as well as representing seniors' political and economic interests. But there are too many people living alone with no social support. If every person, young and old, pledged to honor and care about the plight of older people and people with life-threatening diseases, we can build local social networks across the nation that will enhance quality of life and life expectancy.

Stand up for aging people in America because they are having a difficult time standing up for themselves. Don't let anyone tell you that you don't belong. Public relations campaigns with positive messaging about aging (via television, movies, and radio, print, and social media) are a major step in the right direction. Perhaps more important, these campaigns will create local social networks across America that will lift people's spirits and give them a fighting chance in the battle against aging.

The message is straightforward: Older people are alive and well and have meaning in their lives. Older people have lived long, rewarding lives and they have accumulated wisdom along the way. There is no shame in growing old—older people are proud to be senior citizens. Growing old is a natural and positive process. Aging is beautiful.

United We Age aims to change the way we support and think about older people. The campaign encourages everyone to step up and realize that the solution begins with you. The way older people are seen and judged involves all of us. It means taking responsibility for each other and ourselves.

Visit **www.UnitedWeAge.org**.

Highlights from Profile of Older Americans 2018

(Source: Administration for Community Living, acl.gov/ aging-and-disability-in-america/data-and-research/ profile-older-americans).

About 28 percent (14.3 million) of noninstitutionalized older persons (65+) live alone in the United States today.

Almost half of older women (44 percent) age 75+ live alone.

5 percent of older adults earned income under $15,000 in 2017.

The median income of older persons in 2017 was $32,654 for males and $19,180 for females.

Older persons living alone were much more likely to be poor (16.5 percent) than were older persons living with families (5 percent).

Over the past ten years, the population age 65 and over increased from 37.8 million in 2007 to 50.9 million in 2017 (a 34 percent increase) and is projected to reach 94.7 million in 2060.

The 85 and over population is projected to more than double from 6.5 million in 2017 to 14.4 million in 2040 (34 percent of older adults).

About one in every seven members of the population, or 15.6 percent, is an older American.

Persons reaching age 65 have an average life expectancy of an additional 19.5 years (20.6 years for females and 18.1 years for males).

Older men were much more likely to be married than older women—70 percent of men, 46 percent of women. In 2018, 32 percent of older women were widows.

In 2017, 4.68 million older adults (9.2 percent) were below the poverty level.

The need for caregiving increases with age. From January to June 2018, the percentage of older adults age 85 and over needing help with personal care (20 percent) was more than twice the percentage of adults ages 75-84 (9 percent) and five times the percentage for adults ages 65-74 (4 percent).

In 2017, 23 percent of persons age 65 and over were members of racial or ethnic minority populations—9 percent were African-Americans, 4 percent were Asian, 0.5 percent were American Indian and Alaska Native. Persons of Hispanic origin represented 8 percent of the older population.

Guide to
Key Concepts

There may be instances when you need to refer to one or more of the tasks, activities, or practices presented in this book to help you better cope with an inconvenience of aging, or to better place you on the road to positive aging. Consider this appendix a quick-reference guide—a crib sheet—to the key concepts, tasks, activities, and practices that will lead you to a more joyful life in your twilight years. In addition to defining certain terms, I've provided the number of the chapter where the ideas are discussed most fully.

Acceptance (chapter 6)

Acceptance is one of the keys to stress-free aging.
> ➤ Accept your fate.
> ➤ Be pliable.
> ➤ Accept change.

Adaptation (chapter 6)

Adapting is one of the keys to improving quality of life as you age.

> ➢ Be willing to try new things.
> ➢ Adopt a practical approach to aging.
> ➢ Put quality of life over shame, guilt, and embarrassment.

Affirmations (chapter 5)

Affirmations are suited for applying positivity to help better cope with aging. Here are two of my favorites; see chapter 6, The Four A's, for more affirmations.

> ➢ I am more than my physical body.
> ➢ My spirit strengthens with age.

Age-Induced Depression (chapter 8)

For some of us, the dramatic shift to growing old from youthfulness is emotionally draining, resulting in sadness and perhaps depression. Post meridiem depression is the emotional state (depression) that occurs when we part with our younger selves. Here are some remedies to help us avoid or minimize post meridiem depression:

> ➢ Socialize
> ➢ Maintain structure in your life
> ➢ Continue employment
> ➢ Community service
> ➢ Continuing education

Ageism (chapter 14)

Ageism is the prejudice or discrimination based on a person's age. More specifically, it is discrimination against persons of a certain age group—a tendency to regard older persons as debilitated, unworthy of attention, or unsuitable for employment.

Appreciation (chapter 6)

Appreciation or gratitude is a necessary component to growing old gracefully. Here is how you can practice appreciation:

> ➢ Find pleasure in small things.
> ➢ Be appreciative that you have mobility with a walker, rather than wanting to be able to walk again with no assistance.
> ➢ Keep an appreciation journal, where you write down things for which you are grateful.
> ➢ Wear an appreciation wristband and snap it when you forget to appreciate something in your life.

Attitude (chapter 6)

Aging is all about attitude.

> ➢ Don't cower to those misguided forever-young attitudes that favor the young over the old.
> ➢ Be proud and honored to have lived this long.
> ➢ Have an attitude that older people belong.
> ➢ Have an attitude that older people possess value.
> ➢ Have an attitude that older people are cool.

Balance (chapter 8)

We need to re-balance the composition of our "life" portfolio to better fit the new reality of life as an older person. There are four major categories for balancing as you age:

Lifestyle

> ➢ Eating/diet
> ➢ Healthy choices

➢ Exercise
➢ Activities
➢ Fashion/attire
➢ Organization
➢ Rest

Social Interactions

➢ Participate in group activities.
➢ Learn new skills.
➢ Attend church or other support organizations.
➢ Spend time with family/friends.
➢ Love yourself.
➢ Get out more.

Priorities

➢ Health
➢ Relationships
➢ Purpose
➢ Happiness

Expectations

➢ Expectations prevent you from enjoying the aging experience.
➢ Replace expectations with possibilities and you will be better prepared to deal with aging.

Coping with Mortality (chapter 9)

Many humans cope with mortality by creating beliefs and values that promise a sense of immortality.

➢ Leave a social legacy.
➢ Leave a family legacy.

> ➢ Find meaning in life.
> ➢ Traditional religion
> ➢ New Age beliefs
> ➢ Eastern religious beliefs
> ➢ Accept and appreciate life.

Crystals (chapter 3)

For purposes of tapping into our spirit, believers should use crystals as an aid. For nonbelievers, there may still be a positive psychological effect of using crystals: thinking that maybe they have the power to tap into your spirit.

If you acquire a crystal, put it into practice by wearing it as jewelry, placing it in your home, or carrying it in your pocket. Here are five crystals associated with facilitating a spiritual journey:

Clear Quartz. Quartz is one of the most basic crystals for beginning your spiritual journey. Quartz carries the power to cleanse your thoughts and clear your mind. Once you feel connected to your quartz, clarify your intentions for the stone and trust that it is listening.

Selenite. This stone is known for unblocking stagnant energies, ensuring a positive flow of vibrations between you and your crystals. Selenite is one of the most powerful tools for removing negativity as you age.

Shungite. This stone contains natural antioxidants, making it a powerful healer of health-hazardous energies to the body. It can be used for detoxification and relief from anxiety as you age.

Amethyst. It is believed that this stone acts as an energetic shield containing a spiritual light around your body. This stone is particularly useful for people confronting physical and mental decline because it helps strengthen your spiritual body as well as boosting your self-worth.

Citrine. This stone carries the energy of the sun and promotes happiness and positivity as we cope with the marks of aging. Citrine is a useful crystal for people aging because it fills you with optimism and motivates you to form good habits for life balancing.

Ego (chapter 3)

An untamed ego is your spirit's greatest enemy. Like a jealous 6-year old boy trying to gain the attention of his parents over his 3-year old sister, the ego steps in front of the spirit at every opportunity. Taming your ego is a mandatory first step in tapping into your spirit. You begin by becoming aware that your ego heavily influences your thoughts and actions and that your ego makes it more difficult to age gracefully. Then you will realize that you are in control of your thoughts—not your ego. Do not rush the process; your objective is to make a little progress each day at taming your ego.

Emotional Intelligence (chapter 12)

Wikipedia defines emotional intelligence (EI) as the capability of individuals to recognize their own emotions and those of others, discern different feelings and label them appropriately, use emotional information to guide thinking and behavior, and manage or adjust emotions to adapt to environments or achieve one's goals.

Healthy Habits (chapter 11)

We can't slow down the aging process, but we can avoid aging too quickly.

➤ Simplify your life.
➤ Get enough sleep.
➤ Keep structure in your life.
➤ Practice proper posture.

➤ Stop sitting all the time.
➤ Avoid dry air.
➤ Take Omega-3 fatty acids and take care of your skin complexion.
➤ Take care of yourself.

Healthy Nutrition (chapter 11)

Here are the essential nutrients for seniors as the age:

➤ Vitamin A, B (especially B12), C, D and E
➤ Calcium
➤ Fiber
➤ Protein
➤ Potassium
➤ Magnesium
➤ Zinc

Inconveniences of Aging (chapter 9)

If you live long enough, you will encounter a long and varied list of "inconveniences" due to physical and mental decline. The inconveniences of aging are the marks of aging that we encounter as we grow older. How you prepare for and battle each inconvenience (e.g., disease, hearing impairment, mobility problems) is what determines the quality of your life, both physically and emotionally. Here are the categories of the inconveniences of aging.

➤ Diseases/Conditions
➤ Mental Health
➤ Bodily Functions
➤ Physical Appearance

Meditation (chapter 4)

Meditation is a practice that promotes relaxation, builds internal energy (or life-force) and develops compassion, love, kindness, and an overall sense of well-being. Meditation is perhaps the most effective practice of spirituality. It involves focusing on an object, a point in space, or a mantra (in Buddhist or yoga practices). Some physicians and health centers now routinely recommend meditation or yoga and include them as part of integrated health programs.

When you achieve a deep meditative state, I believe you have touched your spirit.

For people who do not want to fully integrate meditation into their lives, I suggest meditating two times per day for just 2 to 5 minutes in each session.

Morning Meditation. Take 2 to 5 minutes out of your morning to meditate. Morning meditation awakens your spirit, putting you in the best possible position to deal with aging-related issues throughout the day.

Evening Meditation. Take 2 to 5 minutes out of your evening to meditate. Evening meditation helps cleanse your ego's negative thoughts that have built up throughout the day.

Mindfulness (chapter 4)

One of the secrets to successful aging is to live in the present moment with passion and humor. To accomplish this, we practice mindfulness. Mindfulness means living in the moment and awakening to experience.

To attain mindfulness, you should aspire to 30-minute meditation sessions. The more you meditate, the easier it becomes to maintain awareness of your breathing, which helps empty the mind. (See Meditation, above.) Ways to live in the present moment:

➢ Avoid multitasking.
➢ Practice tai chi or qigong.
➢ Block out past thoughts.
➢ Don't worry about the future.

Out-of-Body Experience (chapter 3)

Here is how I experienced an OBE using the Monroe Hemi Sync method:

➢ Lie in bed with hands at your side and get as comfortable as you can. You need to place yourself in the best position and environment to achieve success. And you need to be in a distraction-free environment, where you can darken the room and remain undisturbed during this 30-to-45-minute exercise. Loosen any tight clothing and remove shoes and glasses (or contacts).
➢ You will hear a voice on the Hemi Sync CD, followed by sounds. There are three steps that you must follow for any OBE exercise: create an energy conversion box; cite your affirmation; and conduct resonant tuning.
➢ An energy conversion box is symbolic of a place for you to place all your worries and concerns, leaving you free and unencumbered. Create it in your mind, even if you don't see, hear, or feel it.
➢ Say the affirmation: "I am more than my physical body." The affirmation helps you focus your attention on what you want to accomplish during any exercise. It helps you focus your intent, thereby enabling you to become more aware of your expanding consciousness.
➢ The final step is resonant tuning, which is a breathing exercise to help you vitalize and charge your entire system. It promotes an accelerated gathering of your vibrational energy while reducing your internal dialogue. You will hear strange, eerie sounds of a

symphonic or synthesized nature. You need to put your mind into the rhythmic sound waves.

➢ If you are successful (and it may take three to ten exercises to get there), you will feel a tingling sensation throughout your body. When you do, keep your mind focused and soon the tingling will change into vibrations that will get more intense by the second, capturing your entire body, head to toe.

➢ And then it could happen—you will be looking down at your body. You will have experienced an OBE. It is possible that you will have a sensation that your spirit is floating freely and drifting upward toward the bedroom ceiling. It will be a glorious feeling.

Positive Aging Activities (chapter 12)

Positive aging activities help us maintain a happy and healthy lifestyle and allow us to feel good about ourselves as we experience physical and mental decline. Here are eight task areas that offer a host of activities that will help us age successfully.

➢ Discover and Learn
➢ Fill a Hope Bucket
➢ Do Happy Things
➢ Seize Change
➢ Make a Difference
➢ Bio Legacies
➢ Get to Know People
➢ Sounding Off

Positivity (chapter 5)

Applying positivity to the challenges of aging is straightforward. Negativity can keep older people from truly living life. You can transform your life by staying positive. You need to feel good about yourself no matter what age or mark of aging is challenging you. Here are some habits that you can integrate into your daily life that will help you practice positivity.

- ➢ Saying affirmations (see Affirmations, above)
- ➢ Keeping religious/supernatural beliefs
- ➢ Putting yourself in a happy place
- ➢ Focusing on something positive
- ➢ Keeping a gratitude journal
- ➢ Calming your body

Social Support (chapters 2 and 7)

We must try to maintain or build social networks in our senior years. Without the support of family and friends, quality of life and life expectancy are compromised.

There are numerous ways to ensure that you will have a social support network as you age:

Family

The most effective way of ensuring social support in your senior years is to maintain close and loving relations with family, particularly your children and siblings.

Friends

Maintaining friend relations will serve as a support network as you encounter the marks of aging.

There are a number of ways to meet new friends:

- ➢ Live in a 55+ community.
- ➢ Participate in activities: hiking, dining, yoga classes.
- ➢ Join a fitness center or a senior center that plans activities.

> ➤ Join a bowling league or play golf or tennis.
> ➤ Participate in cards or other group games.
> ➤ Go on group travel trips.

Church and Other Support Organizations

Church is a great place to find support groups for older people. You can also join Internet support groups related to your health concerns (e.g., hearing impairment, dementia).

Tap into Local Organizations/Communities

You can contact local organizations that cater to older people with needs (e.g., Meals on Wheels). Or you can move to a 55+ community or an independent/assisting living facility.

United We Age

There are support groups like United We Age that offer "Friends for Seniors" services, providing social support to people living alone with no support network.

Spirit (chapter 3)

Your spirit is your best friend. It is part of your social group—it's the power of me. As humans age, the physical body declines while the spiritual body continues to grow. Embrace your spiritual body and you will perceive aging through a stronger lens with greater clarity. You will be more confident and secure, and you will no longer be embarrassed or ashamed about marks of aging, whether it's battling cancer or heart disease, a decline in physical appearance, a disabled body function, or a mental impairment. Here are ways to tap into your spirit:

➢ Seeking peaceful moments
➢ Meditation (see Meditation, above)
➢ Out-of-Body Experience (see Out-of-Body Experience, above)
➢ Crystals (see Crystals, above)
➢ Prayer
➢ Yoga
➢ Mind stimulation (drawing; music; writing; reading; mind games)
➢ Love (The more you love yourself (self-love), the closer you are to your spirit.)

United We Age (chapter 16)

If you are fortunate enough to have a family/friend support network, you are well on your way toward positive aging. But there are people aging alone who have little or no social support. Without the help of others, quality of life suffers. I founded United We Age to:

➢ Inspire a movement where the younger generations are more aware and supportive of people aging.
➢ Inspire a movement to build local social support networks across the nation to support people facing quality-of-life decline due to aging, especially people living alone.
➢ Inspire a movement that affects changes in cultural beliefs and attitudes to make America a more age-friendly nation.
➢ www.UnitedWeAge.org

Information Sources for Practicing Positive Aging

There is an abundance of resources available to help you practice positive aging. You just need to know where to look because there is so much out there. The Internet is filled with a plethora of information, research, support groups, tools, and ideas to facilitate positive aging.

My objective is to provide people facing the challenges of aging with the information sources that can aid them better cope with quality-of-life decline due to aging. The sources of information are divided into six categories:

➤ Age-Related Disease and Conditions
➤ Organizations Dedicated to Aging Issues
➤ Aging Research
➤ Online Support Groups
➤ Blogs and Podcasts on Aging Issues
➤ Social Support Organizations

Age-Related Disease and Conditions

Below are sources of information on age-related disease and conditions that you can access. In most cases, you can visit these sources and gather information about your particular mark of aging (e.g., hearing impairment) to gain a fuller understanding of its impact on your health, as well as learn about its symptoms and treatment options

Alliance for Aging Research

Visit this site and learn about the latest information and resources about age-related conditions, diseases, and issues that affect the health of older Americans. Health topics include many of the marks of aging from A to Z (from Age-Related Macular Degeneration to Valve Disease). www.agingresearch.org/health-topic

WebMD

WebMD is a leading source for timely health and medical news and information. The site offers comprehensive information about most of the marks of aging, including disease and illnesses, bodily functions, mental health, and physical decline. www.webmd.com/a-to-z-guides/common-topics.

Mayo Clinic

The Mayo Clinic is an American not-for-profit organization and an academic medical center based in Rochester, Minnesota, focused on integrated clinical practice, education, and research. Visit the Find Diseases & Conditions page to access pertinent information about your particular mark of aging. www.mayoclinic.org

National Institute of Health

Offers studies/research and education on all medical treatment issues—diseases, physical changes, bodily functions, and mental health. www.nih.gov/health-information

Cleveland Clinic

Cleveland Clinic is a nonprofit academic medical center providing clinical and hospital care and is a leader in research, education, and health information. Visit the Cleveland Clinic home page to find an alphabetical listing covering all medical conditions. www.cleveland-clinic.org

National Nonprofit Disease Organizations

American Diabetes Association

The American Diabetes Association is leading the fight against the deadly consequences of diabetes and fighting for those affected by diabetes. The Association funds research to prevent, cure, and manage diabetes; delivers services to hundreds of communities; provides objective and credible information; and gives voice to those denied their rights because of diabetes. Founded in 1940, its mission is to prevent and cure diabetes and to improve the lives of all people affected by diabetes. www.diabetes.org

American Heart Association

The American Heart Association is a national voluntary health agency whose mission is: "Building healthier lives, free of cardiovascular diseases and stroke." www.heart.org

American Kidney Fund

The mission of the American Kidney Fund is to fight kidney disease through direct financial support to patients in need; health education; and prevention efforts. The American Kidney Fund was founded in 1971 to save the life of one person who needed help paying for dialysis. Forty-nine years later, AKF has become the leading source of direct, treatment-related financial assistance to people in the United States who are living with chronic kidney disease. www.kidneyfund.org

American Liver Foundation

The American Liver Foundation was created in 1976 by the American Association for the Study of Liver Disease (AASLD). This organization of scientists and health-care professionals was concerned with the rising incidence of liver disease and the lack of awareness among both the general public and the medical community. The mission, the programs and the services provided by ALF complement the great work of AASLD. The American Liver Foundation's mission is to facilitate, advocate, and promote education, support, and research for the prevention, treatment, and cure of liver disease. www.liverfoundation.org

American Lung Association

The mission of the American Lung Association is to save lives by improving lung health and preventing lung disease. Now in its second century, the American Lung Association is the leading organization working to save lives, improve lung health, and prevent lung disease. www.lung.org

Arthritis Foundation

The mission of the Arthritis Foundation is to improve lives through leadership in the prevention, control, and cure of arthritis and related diseases. The foundation helps people take control of arthritis by providing public health education; pursuing public policy and legislation; and conducting evidence-based programs to improve the quality of life for those living with arthritis. www.arthritis.org

Crohn's and Colitis Foundation of America

The Crohn's and Colitis Foundation of America is a nonprofit, volunteer-driven organization dedicated to finding the cure for Crohn's disease and ulcerative colitis. Today, the Foundation funds cutting-edge studies at major medical institutions, nurtures investigators at the early stages of their careers, and finances underdeveloped areas of research. Educational workshops and symposia, together with its scientific journal, *Inflammatory Bowel Diseases*, enable medical professionals to keep pace with this rapidly growing field. www.crohnscolitisfoundation.org

Cystic Fibrosis Foundation

The mission of the Cystic Fibrosis Foundation, a nonprofit donor-supported organization, is to ensure the development of the means to cure and control cystic fibrosis and to improve the quality of life for those with the disease. The Foundation is the leading organization in the United States devoted to cystic fibrosis. It funds and accredits more than 115 CF care centers, 95 adult care programs, and 50 affiliate programs, and has 80 chapters and branch offices nationwide. www.cff.org

Depression and Bipolar Support Alliance

The Depression and Bipolar Support Alliance (DBSA) is the leading patient-directed national organization focusing on the most prevalent mental illnesses. The organization fosters an environment of understanding about the impact and management of these life-threatening illnesses by providing up-to-date, scientifically based tools and information written in language the general public can understand. www.dbsalliance.org

Hearing Loss Association of America

The Hearing Loss Association of America (HLAA) is the nation's leading organization representing consumers with hearing loss. www.hearingloss.org

Muscular Dystrophy Association

MDA is the nonprofit health agency dedicated to curing muscular dystrophy, ALS, and related diseases by funding worldwide research. The Association also provides comprehensive health care and support services, advocacy, and education. www.mda.org

National Alliance on Mental Illness

From its inception in 1979, NAMI has been dedicated to improving the lives of individuals and families affected by mental illness. www.nami.org

Arthritis Foundation

The Arthritis Foundation is the only national not-for-profit organization that supports the more than 100 types of arthritis and related conditions. www.arthritis.org

National Brain Tumor Society

The National Brain Tumor Society is a nonprofit organization inspiring hope and providing leadership within the brain tumor community. It exists to find a cure and improve the quality of life for those affected by brain tumors. www.braintumor.org

National Breast Cancer Foundation

The National Breast Cancer Foundation's mission is to save lives by increasing awareness of breast cancer through education and by providing mammograms for those in need. www.Nationalbreastcancer.org

National Lung Cancer Partnership

The National Lung Cancer Partnership (formerly Women Against Lung Cancer) is a nonprofit organization, originally formed in 2001. Its mission is to decrease deaths due to lung cancer, and help patients live longer and better, through research, awareness, and advocacy. www.nationallungcancerpartnership.org

National Osteoporosis Foundation

The mission of the National Osteoporosis Foundation is to prevent osteoporosis and related fractures, to promote lifelong bone health, to help improve the lives of those affected by osteoporosis, and to find a cure through programs of awareness, advocacy, public and health professional education, and research. www.nof.org

National Sleep Foundation

The National Sleep Foundation (NSF) is a nonprofit organization dedicated to improving public health and safety by achieving understanding of sleep and sleep disorders, and by supporting sleep-related education, research, and advocacy. www.sleepfoundation.org

Sickle Cell Disease Association of America

The association advocates for and enhances membership's ability to improve the quality of health, life, and services for individuals, families, and communities affected by sickle cell disease and related conditions, while promoting the search for a cure for all people in the world with sickle cell disease. www.sicklecelldisease.org

Pulmonary Fibrosis Foundation

The Pulmonary Fibrosis Foundation is a nonprofit organization founded in 2001 to accelerate research efforts leading to a cure for pulmonary fibrosis (PF), while educating, supporting, and advocating for the community of patients, families, and medical professionals fighting this disease. www.coalitionforpf.org

Leukemia & Lymphoma Society

The Leukemia & Lymphoma Society (LLS) is the world's largest voluntary health organization dedicated to funding blood cancer research, education, and patient services. LLS's mission: Cure leukemia, lymphoma, Hodgkin's disease, and myeloma, and improve the quality of life of patients and their families. www.lls.org

National Multiple Sclerosis Society

The National Multiple Sclerosis Society is a collective of passionate individuals who want to do something about MS now—to move together toward a world free of multiple sclerosis. www.nationalmssociety.org

Vasculitis Foundation

The Vasculitis Foundation advocates for early diagnosis, leading-edge treatment, and ultimately a cure for all types of vasculitis. The Vasculitis Foundation supports and empowers patients through education, awareness, and research. www.vasculitisfoundation.org

Organizations Dedicated to Aging Issues

Below are some organizations dedicated to aging issues. These organizations are committed to helping people live longer and happier lives.

Professional Organizations

American Society on Aging

This organization links all sorts of professionals dedicated to elderly care through conferences, professional education, awards, and journals. www.asaging.org

Academy for Gerontology in Higher Education

Through the participation of its member institutions, a quarterly newsletter, and an annual conference, this organization brings together academics in the field of gerontology from many different colleges and universities. www.aghe.org

The Gerontological Society of America

This professional organization aims to improve and disseminate the latest aging research to doctors, scientists, and policymakers. www.geron.org

Public Awareness Organizations

National Council on Aging

A leading nonprofit advocating for America's elderly, this group supports both health and economic security for old people in the United States. www.ncoa.org

American Association of Retired Persons (AARP)

AARP is a nonprofit, nonpartisan organization with a membership that helps people 50+ have independence, choice, and control in ways that are beneficial and affordable to them and society as a whole. www.aarp.org

RRF Foundation for Aging

Through numerous small grants, this organization aims to raise the quality of life for America's elderly population. It does this by supporting greater autonomy and status in society. www.rrf.org

Methuselah Foundation

The lofty goal of this charity is making 90-year-olds as healthy as 50-year-olds by 2030. A goal it hopes to reach through fundraising for research in the exciting field of regenerative medicine. www.mfoundation.org

The Commonwealth Fund

With an endowment of roughly $700 million, this foundation has been working to improve health care for vulnerable populations since 1918, with many programs aimed at elderly adults. www.commonwealthfund.org/about-us

Leadership Council of Aging Organizations

The Leadership Council of Aging Organizations (LCAO) is a coalition of national nonprofit organizations concerned with the well-being of America's older population and committed to representing their interests in the policymaking arena. www.lcao.org/about-lcao/membership. The following organizations are members of LCAO and whose missions are consistent with the practice of positive aging.

AASC

The American Association of Service Coordinators is a national nonprofit dedicated to advance the interests of the Service Coordinator profession and provide guidance and professional standards to members. AASC's vision is to support its members that serve individuals, families, the elderly, and persons with disabilities in hous-ing situations through leadership, education, training, networking, advocacy, and other member services. www.servicecoordinator.org

Aging Life Care Association

Aging Life Care—a holistic, client-centered approach to caring for older adults or others facing ongoing health challenges. Working with families, the expertise of Aging Life Care Professionals provides the answers at a time of uncertainty. www.aginglifecare.org

Alliance for Aging Research

The Alliance for Aging Research is the leading nonprofit organization dedicated to accelerating the pace of scientific discoveries and their application to vastly improve the universal human experience of aging and health. www.agingresearch.org

Alliance for Retired Americans

The mission of the Alliance for Retired Americans is to ensure social and economic justice and full civil rights for all citizens so that they may enjoy lives of dignity, personal and family fulfillment, and secu-rity. retiredamericans.org

Alzheimer's Association

The Alzheimer's Association is the leading global voluntary health organization in Alzheimer care and support, and the largest private, nonprofit funder of Alzheimer research. www.alz.org

American Geriatrics Society

The American Geriatrics Society (AGS) is a not-for-profit organi-zation of over 6,000 health professionals dedicated to improving the health, independence, and quality of life of older people through initiatives in patient care, research, professional and public education, and public policy. www.americangeriatrics.org

AMDA – The Society for Post-Acute and Long-Term Care Medicine

AMDA – The Society for Post-Acute and Long-Term Care Medicine is the only medical specialty society representing the community of over 50,000 medical directors, physicians, nurse practitioners, physician assistants, and other practitioners working in the various post-acute and long-term care (PA/LTC) settings. The Society's 5,500 members work in skilled nursing facilities, long-term care and assisted living communities, CCRCs, home care, hospice, PACE programs, and other settings. www.paltc.org

American Society on Aging (ASA)

The American Society on Aging is an association of diverse individuals bound by a common goal: to support the commitment and enhance the knowledge and skills of those who seek to improve the quality of life of older adults and their families. www.asaging.org

Association of Jewish Aging Services (AJAS)

AJAS is a unique association of not-for-profit community-based organizations, rooted in Jewish values, which promotes and supports the delivery of services to an aging population. www.ajas.org

Caring Across Generations

Caring Across Generations brings together aging Americans, people with disabilities, workers, and their families to protect all Americans' right to choose the care and support they need to live with dignity. www.caringacross.org

Center for Medicare Advocacy. (CMA)

The Center for Medicare Advocacy's mission is to advance access to comprehensive Medicare coverage and quality health care for older people and people with disabilities by providing exceptional analysis, education, and advocacy. www.medicareadvocacy.org

Compassion & Choices

Compassion & Choices is the leading nonprofit organization committed to helping everyone have the best death possible. It offers free consultation, planning resources, referrals, and guidance, and across the nation works to protect and expand options at the end of life. www.compassionandchoices.org

Experience Works

Improve the lives of older people through training, community service, and employment. www.experienceworks.org.

The Gerontological Society of America

The Gerontological Society of America's (GSA) mission is to advance the study of aging and disseminate information among scientists, decision-makers, and the general public. www.geron.org

Justice in Aging

Justice in Aging uses the power of law and its expertise in government safety-net programs like Medicare, Medicaid, Social Security, and SSI to fight senior poverty. The organization engages in three main arenas to protect the rights of poor seniors and strengthen the programs they rely on: administrative advocacy, providing expertise and resources to direct service advocates, and litigation. justiceinaging.org

LeadingAge

The mission of LeadingAge is to be the trusted voice for aging in America. Its 6,000+ members and partners include not-for-profit organizations representing the entire field of aging services, 39 state partners, hundreds of businesses, consumer groups, foundations, and research partners. LeadingAge is also a part of The Global Ageing Network (formerly IAHSA), whose membership spans 30 countries. LeadingAge is a 501I(3) tax-exempt charitable organization focused on education, advocacy and applied research. www.leadingage.org

Meals on Wheels America

Meals On Wheels America is the oldest and largest membership organization supporting the national network of more than 5,000 Senior Nutrition Programs that operate in all 50 states and U.S. territories. www.mealsonwheelsamerica.org

Medicare Rights Center

The Medicare Rights Center is a national, nonprofit consumer service organization that works to ensure access to affordable health care for older adults and people with disabilities through counseling and advocacy, educational programs, and public policy initiatives. www.medicarerights.org

National Academy of Elder Law Attorneys (NAELA)

The mission of the National Academy of Elder Law Attorneys is to establish NAELA members as the premier providers of legal advocacy, guidance, and services to enhance the lives of people with special needs and people as they age. www.naela.org

National Adult Protective Services Association (NAPSA)

The goal of the National Adult Protective Services Association (NAPSA), formed in 1989, is to provide Adult Protective Services (APS) programs, a forum for sharing information, solving problems, and improving the quality of services for victims of elder and vulnerable adult mistreatment. www.napsa-now.org

National Alliance for Caregiving

The National Alliance for Caregiving is a nonprofit coalition of national organizations—including grassroots organizations, professional associations, service organizations, disease-specific organizations, a government agency, and corporations—focusing on issues of family caregiving. www.caregiving.org

National Asian Pacific Center on Aging (NAPCA)

The National Asian Pacific Center on Aging is the nation's leading advocacy and service organization committed to the dignity, well-being, and quality of life of Asian American and Pacific Islanders as they age. (napca.org)

National Association for Home Care & Hospice (NAHC)

The National Association for Home Care & Hospice (NAHC) is the largest and most respected professional association representing the interests of chronically ill, disabled, and dying Americans of all ages and the caregivers who provide them with in-home health and hospice services. www.nahc.org

National Association of Area Agencies on Aging (n4a)

The National Association of Area Agencies on Aging (n4a) is a 501c(3) membership association representing America's national network of more than 600 Area Agencies on Aging (AAAs) and providing a voice in the nation's capital for the 250+ Title VI Native American aging programs. www.n4a.org

National Association of Nutrition and Aging Services Programs (NANASP)

NANASP is an organization of over 1,100 national advocates for senior health and well-being who strengthen the policies and programs that nourish seniors. www.nanasp.org

National Association of State Ombudsman Programs (NASOP)

As mandated by the Older Americans Act, the mission of the Long-Term Care Ombudsman Program is to seek resolution of problems and advocate for the rights of residents of long-term care facilities, with the goal of enhancing the quality of life and care of residents. www.nasop.org

ADvancing States

ADvancing States represents the nation's fifty-six state and territorial agencies on aging and disabilities and supports visionary state leadership, the advancement of state systems innovation, and the articulation of national policies that support home and community-based services for older adults and individuals with disabilities. www.nasuad.org

National Caucus and Center for Black Aging, Inc. (NCBA)

NCBA is one of the country's oldest organizations dedicated to aging issues and the only national organization devoted to minority and low-income aging. www.ncba-aged.org

National Center for Creative Aging

The National Center for Creative Aging (NCCA) is dedicated to fostering an understanding of the vital relationship between creative expression and healthy aging, and to developing programs that build upon this understanding. It works on all facets of aging to build a world where all individuals flourish across their life span through creative expression. www.creativeaging.org

The National Consumer Voice for Quality Long-Term Care

The Consumer Voice is a leading national organization representing consumers in issues related to long-term care, helping to ensure that consumers are empowered to advocate for themselves. theconsumervoice.org

National Council on Aging (NCOA)

Founded in 1950, the National Council on Aging (NCOA) is the first national nonprofit representing older adults and the community organizations that serve them; its mission is to improve the lives of millions of older adults, especially those who are struggling. www.ncoa.org

National Hispanic Council on Aging (NHCOA)

The National Hispanic Council on Aging (NHCOA) is the premier nonprofit organization in the nation advocating on behalf of Hispanic older adults. www.nhcoa.org

National Indian Council on Aging (NICOA)

The National Indian Council On Aging, Inc. (NICOA), a nonprofit organization, was founded in 1976 by members of the National Tribal Chairmen's Association, which called for a national organization focused on aging American Indian and Alaska Native Elders. nicoa. org

Visiting Nurse Associations of America (VNAA)

VNAA supports, promotes, and advances nonprofit providers of community-based health care, including home health, hospice, and palliative care, and health promotion services to ensure quality care within their communities. www.vnaa.org

Aging Research

Below are journals dedicated to aging research that do not require a subscription. www.publichealth.org/resources/aging

Geriatrics & Gerontology International

The official journal of the Japan Geriatrics Society, this quarterly publishes multidisciplinary aging research particularly relevant to societies with growing elderly populations.

Frontiers in Aging Neuroscience

This open-access Swiss publication focuses on understanding the fundamental processes behind Alzheimer's and other age-related diseases. www.frontiersin.org/journals/aging-neuroscience

Aging

This journal covers recent discoveries on the aging process from the molecular to the human level. www.impactaging.com.

Research Organizations

Below are some of the top research organizations dedicated to making life longer and happier.

The Larry Ellison Foundation

This nonprofit organization supports scholarly research that sets out to understand the fundamentals of the aging process. The website features an informative overview covering its major aging-related research areas. www.ellisonfoundation.org

Cancer & Aging Research Group

Cancer is the second most common killer of elderly Americans. This organization aims to bring together researchers from across the country through grants and ongoing studies on cancer treatment. www.mycarg.org

The Dartmouth Institute for Health Policy and Clinical Practice

This research institute focuses on improving clinical practice and health policy for older Americans. www.tdi.dartmouth.edu/research

Albert Einstein College of Medicine Institute for Aging Research

The Albert Einstein College of Medicine has a reputation for cutting-edge medical research, and the Aging Institute focuses particularly on understanding the genetics of growing old and extending human life. www.einstein.yu.edu/centers/aging

Institute on Aging

This research institute at the University of Pennsylvania School of Medicine gives particular attention to treating neurocognitive diseases like Alzheimer's. www.med.upenn.edu/aging

Buck Institute for Research on Aging

The oldest independent research facility in the United States dedicated exclusively to aging, this organization focuses on understanding and treating common old-age afflictions like cancer, stroke, Alzheimer's, and Parkinson's disease. www.buckinstitute.org

Institute for Aging ResearchHebrew SeniorLife

Affiliated with Harvard University, this Boston-based facility is the largest gerontological research center in the United States, developing new treatments for old-age brain and bone health. www.hebrewseniorlife.org

American Federation for Aging Research

Since its start in 1981, this independent foundation has provided well over $100 million to biomedical researchers working to understand the fundamentals of the aging process. www.afar.org

UCLA Longevity Center

Based at one of the top universities for geriatric medicine in the United States, the UCLA Longevity Center aims to develop new treatments and approaches for elderly care. www.semel.ucla.edu/longevity

Selective Books
Related to Positive Aging

How to Live Forever: The Enduring Power of Connecting the Generations,
by Mark Freedman (Public Affairs Publishers, November, 2018)

Life Reimagined: Discovering Your New Life Possibilities, by Richard
Leider and Alan Webber (Berrett Koehler Publishers, October
2013)

Great Jobs for Everyone 50+, by Kerry Hannon (John Wiley & Sons,
2012)

The Encore Career Handbook, by Marci Alboher (Workman Publishing, 2013)

The Mature Mind: The Positive Power of the Aging Brain, by Gene D.
Cohen (Basic Books, 2005)

Selective Research Articles
Related to Positive Aging

"Positive Aging: New Images for a New Age," MM Gergen, KJ Gergen, Ageing International, 2001, Google: Positive Aging: New
Images for a New Age

"Self Compassion: A Resource for Positive Aging," WJ Phillips, SJ
Ferguson, *Journals of Gerontology* Series B, 2013,

"Growing Older Without Aging? Positive Aging, Anti-Ageism, and
Anti-Aging," S Katz, *Generations* 25(4):27-32, 2001, Researchgate.net

"A Positive Aging Framework for Guiding Geropsychology Interventions," RD Hill, *Behavior Therapy*, 2001, Elsevier

"Quality of Life, Life Satisfaction, and Positive Aging," R Fernandez-Ballesteros, A Kruse, *Aging World*, 2007.

"Ways of Aging," JF Gubrium, JA Holstein, 2008, books.goggle.com.

"Gerotranscendence: A Developmental Theory of Positive Aging,"
Lars Tornstam, Springer Publishing Company, NY, 2005.

"Handbook of Communication and Aging Research," JF Nussbaum,

J Coupland, 2004, books.google.com.

"And as I Go, I Love to Sing: The Happy Wanderers, Music and Positive Aging," JE Southcott, *International Journal of Community Music*, 2009

"Embodying Positive Aging and Neoliberal Rationality: Talking about the Aging Body within Narratives of Retirement," DL Rudman, *Journal of Aging Studies*, 2015, Elservier.

"Solutionism, the Game: Design Fictions for Positive Aging," M Blythe, J Steane, J Roe, C Oliver, Proceedings of the 33rd Annual, ACM Conference on Human Factors in Computing Systems, 2015, dl.acm.org

"Reducing Cardiovascular Stress with Positive Self-Stereotypes of Aging," BR Levy, JM Hausdorff, R Hencke, *The Journals of Gerontology*: Series B, Volume 55, Issue 4, July 1, 2000. Academic.oup. com.

"Another Wrinkle in the Debate about Successful Aging: The Undervalued Concept of Resilience and the Lived Experience of Dementia," PB Harris, *The International Journal of Aging and Human Development*, 2008, journals.sagepub.com.

"Smart Homes for Older People: Positive Aging in a Digital World," Q Le, HB Nguyen, T Barnett, Future Internet, 2012, mdpi.com.

"The Concepts of Successful and Positive Aging," A Bowling, *Family Practice*, 1993, Academic.oup.com.

"Contemporary Issues in Gerontology: Promoting Positive Aging," V Minishiello, I Coulson, Routledge Publishers, September 2005.

"Positive Aging: A Critical Analysis," J Davey, K Glasgow, *Policy Quarterly*, 2006, ojs.victoria.ac.nz

"Positive Ageing, Objective, Subjective and Combined Outcomes," R Fernandez-Ballesteros-Sensoria, *A Journal of Mind, Brain & Education*, 2001, researchgate.net

Online Support Groups

There is an abundance of online support groups for senior citizens; you just have to find the right one for you. There are support groups for most marks of aging (e.g., arthritis), as well as support groups for spirituality. Joining a support group is easy; just Google the type of support group you wish to join, and a list of groups will appear in your geographic location.

Many of the large aging organizations offer online support groups on a variety of topics. These include WebMD, Mayo Clinic, National Institute of Health, Healthfinder.gov, World Health Organization, and Facebook.

Mayo Clinic: online support groups: www.mayoclinic.org/healthy-lifestyle/stress-management/in-depth/support-groups/art-20044655

World Health Organization: search for support groups: patient support groups by country www.who.int/genomics/public/patientsupport/en/

Health Finder.gov (U.S. Department of Health and human Services): healthfinder.gov

WebMD, www.WebMd.com

Facebook, Groups for seniors: Log into your Facebook profile; in the left column, under the Explore heading, click on Groups. Click on the Discover tab at the top of the page. Facebook will bring up some recommended groups based on Pages you've liked. You can also scroll through various topics – like – Seniors, to find relevant groups.

Below is a sample of other useful online support groups for you to join. Again, Google "online support groups for older people" to identify the right group in your local area.

Peer Spirit Circles

Helping people use the circle process in creating the environment for sustaining conversation about proactive, productive aging. www.passitonnetwork.org

Spirituality Support Group

www.managedhealthcareconnect.com/articles/spirituality-and-aging-support-groups-psycho-spiritual-intervention-address-mental-health

Senior Health & Aging Support Group

www.dailystrength.org/group/senior-health-aging

Dementia Caregivers Support Group

www.facebook.com/groups/1516449868588963/?ref=br_rs
Seniors Daily Strength: Issues of concern to seniors, including Alzheimer's, arthritis, osteoporosis, and depression, www.dailystrength.org/categories/Seniors

Blogs and Podcasts on Aging Issues

Many blogs and podcasts on aging issues are useful because they are updated regularly, have a substantial following, and encourage a positive approach to aging. Google "blogs or podcasts on aging issues" and a long list will appear. Here are just a handful.

Feedspot's Top 60 Aging Blogs & Websites for Healthy Aging in 2020. blog.feedspot.com/aging_blogs/

Fight Aging!

Helps you understand the mechanisms behind degenerative aging, and work toward preventing these types of diseases. www.fightaging.org

The New Old Age

A *New York Times* blog that offers insight into aging issues for those who are older. It's about what makes old age rewarding, and some of the challenges faced by older Americans. newoldage.blogs.nytimes.com

Elder Chicks

A blog focused on senior women in their retirement years. Offers funny and relatable stories about elderly women. www.elderchicks. wordpress.com

Time Goes By

This is a blog about what it's really like to get older. The blog covers social issues, work, retirement, age discrimination and ageism, health and politics, and so on. www.timegoesby.net

Fearless Aging

This is a podcast about why and how to live a long, healthy, fit, energetic, and vital life and never be old at any age. Rico and guests will offer you proven tips for mind, body, and spirit and strategies that will help you resolve most health challenges. The podcast presents one show per month. www.spreaker.com/show/fearless-aging.

Live Long and Master Aging

This is a podcast where Peter Bowes interviews leading longevity scientists and people who have mastered the art of aging; two episodes per month. www.llamapodcast.com.

Social Support Organizations

There are literally thousands of compassionate organizations across the nation established to support older people in need, especially those living alone. Use Google to search for the services you seek in your local area. The following list presents typical services for senior citizens in most local areas of the nation.

- ➤ Home-delivered meals
- ➤ Congregate meals served in a community setting
- ➤ Transportation
- ➤ Personal care
- ➤ Nutrition education/counseling
- ➤ Adult day care
- ➤ Case management of a senior's health care
- ➤ Chore services (e.g., household tasks)
- ➤ Legal assistance
- ➤ Caregiver services

Here is a sample of the types of organizations that offer the services listed above.

United We Age

My own nonprofit organization, United We Age, offers a Friends for Seniors program. The program is designed to befriend on older person who lacks meaningful social support (e.g., family/friends) by visiting them periodically and giving them birthday and holiday cards and gifts. www.unitedweage.org

Northland Foundation

The Northland Foundation offers an Age to Age social support program that links children and youth with older adults to build friendships and work together toward community improvement. This grassroots intergenerational initiative has created a new pathway to bring people 55 and older together with children and youth, as well as the generations in between. www.northlandfdn.org

TTN Caring Collaborative

The TTN Caring Collaborative is the work of a volunteer committee of members. It mobilizes goodwill within TTN's membership to support members when in need. They learn from the health-care experiences of others—what to expect during breast cancer treatment, how to optimize recovery following knee replacement surgery, etc. www.thetransitionnetwork.org

CareInHomes

Provides in-home caregiving services, including bathing, companionship, and non-medical assistance. www.careinhome.com.

Elder Helpers

Currently over 10,000 volunteers are standing by to give back to the community or occupy their free time, in addition to gaining wisdom from being in contact with elders. The organization's services include home care, transportation, and companionship, to name a few. www.elderhelpers.org.

The Adult Activity Center of the Treasure Coast

This company offers adult day care services in a safe and caring environment. Nutritious meals and snacks, nursing services, and activities are included. www.seniordaycareportstlucie.com

Legal Services for Seniors

Legal Services for Seniors provides legal services at no charge to Monterey County seniors 60 years of age and older, with an emphasis on the socially or economically needy. www.lssmc.net

Seniors Helping Seniors

Seniors Helping Seniors offers assistance to other seniors in need with a variety of services to help out around the house. Its providers can help with tasks such as light housekeeping (vacuuming, dusting, cleaning the kitchen and bathrooms, taking out the trash, etc.), meal preparation, organizing and consolidating, dressing, bathing and grooming, as well as medication reminders and mobility assistance. www.homecarebyseniors.com/services/around-the-house

Anatomy of a Cancer Survivor

Note: This appendix presents my excruciating battle with cancer. At times, the battle turned ugly and some of my experiences with medical issues may be offensive and a bit depressing to readers. My objective is to tell the true story about my journey with cancer and to be descriptive when necessary. Reader discretion is advised.

My journey began, in Nashville, Tennessee, at the funeral of my wife's sister, who died of stage 4 plasma cell leukemia. I had experienced modest swallowing problems during meals over the previous year, but I shrugged it off as nothing serious. However, at the reception following the funeral, I struggled mightily swallowing chicken tenders. I told no one, not even my wife.

I surmised that there were two possible causes for my swallowing troubles: dysphagia or esophageal cancer. Dysphagia is a problem with the muscular tube that moves food and liquids from the back of your mouth to your stomach. If it is not dysphagia, it is likely that tumors are blocking the esophagus and the likelihood that the tumors are cancerous is high.

My gut told me I had esophageal cancer. I researched esophageal cancer and discovered that one of the primary causes of the cancer was years of experiencing acid reflux, which I had endured for the past seven to ten years. But as fate would have it, my daughter announced her wedding plans, which included a ceremony and reception in my town of Vero Beach, Florida. I had the pleasurable burden of arranging and hosting my daughter's wedding and I was not going to let esophageal cancer interfere. I kept my condition silent for six months until the wedding bells rang.

A week after the wedding, I had an endoscopy. An endoscopy is a procedure performed by a gastroenterologist to examine the esophagus and stomach using a thin, flexible tube called an upper endoscope through which the lining of the esophagus and stomach can be viewed. After the exam, my gastroenterologist told me I had Barrett's esophagus, which meant tissue in my esophagus had transformed into tissue similar to intestinal lining. Barrett's esophagus is often associated with people who have experienced long-term gastroesophageal reflux (acid). This tissue had several large tumors attached to it that inhibited my ability to swallow. A biopsy was performed to determine whether the tumors were cancerous.

Two days later, the gastroenterologist told my wife and me that the biopsy confirmed I had esophageal cancer. I felt nothing—no sadness, no fear, no emotion. He gave me the names of thoracic oncologists to contact in Vero Beach. I left his office with a blank stare. Although I had suspected cancer all along, I was in utter shock at the reality.

I called my primary doctor to tell her the news and to seek guidance. She recommended that I avoid Vero Beach oncologists and go directly to the Moffitt Cancer Center in Tampa, where they have specialists in esophageal cancer. She also introduced me to Jan, a patient of hers who had battled esophageal cancer at the Moffitt Cancer Center two years earlier.

My conversation with Jan was comforting to me. Just knowing she survived boosted my confidence. However, she also gave me a dose of reality: She had been through hell. The chemotherapy and radiation treatment were very taxing, and the surgery was brutal. Her surgery had been two years prior, and she was still recovering.

On the first morning after I learned that I had esophageal cancer, I walked outside, and the sun had never looked brighter, the trees never looked stronger, and the grass never looked greener.

My battle against cancer began the day I visited the Moffitt Cancer Center. I met with the thoracic oncologist and he had the results of a PET scan (positron emission tomography) in front of him. He was straightforward and blunt with me. I had stage 3 esophageal cancer, including several large cancerous tumors attached to my esophagus and cancer in a nearby lymph node.

Stage 3 esophageal cancer meant tumors had penetrated into but not through my esophagus's muscular wall, and cancer cells were found in lymph nodes but no other organs. The usual approach is a combined attack with radiation, chemotherapy, and surgery.

I was one stage away from certain death. Stage 4 esophageal cancer occurs when the tumors penetrate through the esophagus's muscular wall into the liver or lungs or bones. This is a metastatic state with few treatment options.

The doctor made no promises. He did not offer comforting words like "Don't worry, we'll beat this." It was a surreal experience for me. The doctor told me stage 3 esophageal cancer was life-threatening and he laid out a game plan with no guarantees.

As I left the doctor's office, the nurse looked at me with reassuring eyes and said: "If you survive this—your cancer is an inconvenience." I didn't know at the moment, but she was so on target. Every second, every minute, every day, every week, every month, every year, and every decade we are here in the physical realm we call Earth—we are blessed. This is true for any mark of aging, whether hearing loss, mobility loss, arthritis, Parkinson's disease, Alzheimer's, or multiple sclerosis.

The treatment plan included six weeks of intense chemotherapy and radiation, and if it was successful, I would undergo a seven-hour surgery on my esophagus and stomach. If the treatments was not successful, I would endure more chemotherapy and radiation.

The surgery was an Ivor Lewis esophagectomy, where the esophageal tumors are removed through an abdominal incision and a right thoracotomy (a surgical incision of the chest wall). They would cut my lower esophagus and the upper part of my stomach and then reconnect these vital organs. They would collapse part of my lung during surgery to have room to operate. They would also remove a large number of lymph nodes.

Other than a small risk of death, the primary risks of surgery were pneumonia, infection, and blood clots. Again, the doctor emphasized that this would be the worst, most difficult surgery I would ever experience.

Right after I learned about my treatment plan, I thought back on something Jan told me—that I will be shocked throughout my cancer battle about friends and some family who will step up or will step out of my life. Some people step up to the plate, while others bow out.

My biggest fear was that the chemotherapy and radiation treatment wouldn't work, my cancer would metastasize, my tumors would spread, and I would turn into one of those cancer victims who continually get treatment at different centers with little promise of anything working. This was a worst-case scenario that all cancer victims dread. However, I had a genuine hope of recovery. How did I maintain hope? I really don't know.

I was not under the illusion that some miracle would occur, and I would live happily ever after. I knew that none of us escape the deathly clutch of the Grim Reaper. I just had to learn to accept and live with my fate and situation in life. This was the hand I'd been dealt, and I had to go with it. Every cancer victim finds his or her own way to fight, and I had to find mine.

I had more questions than answers as I began my battle with cancer. Did I possess the courage and determination to endure the hurdles that lay ahead? How long did I have? Could I live a normal life?

Get with the Program

I did not have time to sweat the small stuff. My wife and I went into battle mode with a bunker mentality. We moved into a Marriott Residence Inn in Tampa for the six-week treatment period. I knew that even with the most thorough preparation, the battle against cancer could be fraught with debilitating side effects like emotional fatigue, anxiety, and depression.

I received heavy doses of chemotherapy infusions via a pump and portal in addition to radiation therapy Monday through Friday for six weeks. In the operating room, doctors inserted a port into my upper chest area while I was under anesthesia. One end of a catheter was placed in the subclavian vein and the other end was threaded beneath my skin to create a "port pocket." This gave doctors direct access, via the port connecting to the subclavian vein, to the right atrium of my heart. Chemotherapy drugs were pumped directly into my heart, which distributed them throughout my entire body. What a comforting thought.

They infused the chemotherapy drug (poison) Cisplatin through an intravenous bag directed into the port system, which created two hours of nausea. Then the chemo drug 5FU was administered via a wearable pump (a hollow tube with a balloon). As the balloon deflated throughout the week, milliliters of the 5FU poison entered the port and ultimately my blood stream.

My radiation treatment was at 3:45 p.m. Monday through Friday. I lay still in a form-fitted bed as Trilogy 1 (the radiation device) emitted powerful blasts of radiation; its mission was to destroy (shrink) the tumors in my esophagus.

Six weeks of intense chemotherapy and radiation took their toll on me. I was now a member of the walking wounded at the Moffitt Cancer Center. I wore a chemotherapy pump Monday through Friday infusing poisonous chemotherapy drugs into my portal and blood stream. I was in a constant state of nausea. I gagged at the smell of food and regularly vomited in the mornings.

I felt vulnerable, fragile, and uncomfortable wearing the chemo pump around my waist. I walked into a Walmart and saw healthy people who only worried about backaches, the flu, and arthritis, not death. I stuck out like a sore thumb, at least in my head. Other people were normal, and I was strange.

My lifestyle had changed for the worse and I needed to accept what would eventually become routine. Through it all, my wife stood loyally by my side, and my immediate family (children, siblings, and parents) provided tremendous love and emotional support. Some of our best friends volunteered to watch and care for our home while we were away. I quickly learned the importance of social support in a health crisis.

Quite early in the process, I learned that the most important thing is not how strong my wife was for me—she had her emotional moments. What made the difference is how much love she has for me. It is her love that got me through this, not her strength. There is a big difference.

My favorite activity for coping during my six weeks at the Moffitt Cancer Center was taking daily walks on a tree-lined street next to the Residence Inn. As I walked, I contemplated life and wrote down my thoughts in the Notes application on my iPhone. It was therapeutic.

Here are some of the thoughts that I recorded during those walks:

Don't worry about my cancer to the point that I forget to live. I choose to live each day.

If fear or grief move in on me, I will let those emotions in. Then I need to concentrate on being in the moment, right here and now—with gratitude.

I figured I had 80 years to work on my legacy. Suddenly, everything got magnified. But I still want to figure out my purpose and meaning in life.

Cancer becomes something you live with, perhaps with a renewed focus on finishing life's unfinished business, rather than something you inevitably die from.

I need to think of cancer as something to be managed.

I worry that my cancer will metastasize to my lungs or liver. I need to stop worrying.

When you are young and healthy, you feel bulletproof. Now you feel like what the f—k just happened?

Some mornings on chemo, I just don't want to get out of bed, but that is not the way to go about life.

Life is fleeting, isn't it? Memories flood my thoughts. They almost suffocate my thoughts. I go in and out, wandering from my teenage years to adult years. Most of my memories are pleasant, though—fond remembrances. That's a good thing.

How do I deal with my children? It is one thing for them to support me, but how do I tell them not to worry and it is going to be all right?

Too often cancer patients find themselves fighting alone. I've learned you are better off surrounded by family and friends who want to be there.

I was trying to cope with short-term problems like gagging and vomiting—due to the chemo and radiation treatment. These were temporary because after six weeks the treatment program would come to an end. At some point, I would have to deal with the longer-term implications of my cancer. These would be life-altering changes that would likely result in a significant decline in quality of life.

The Worst Surgery of My Life

A PET scan showed that the chemotherapy and radiation treatment were effective; the cancerous tumors had shrunk substantially, and there were no signs of metastasizing. But I had to wait six more weeks until surgery. I needed time to get healthy again after being infused with the poisonous chemo chemicals and bombarded with radiation.

With my wife by my side, I checked in at 6 a.m. on Friday morning, July 8, 2016, to the Moffitt Cancer Center Hospital to prepare for surgery. My three children and sister gathered around at 9 a.m. in the post-surgery waiting area. Everyone was anxious, including yours truly.

My wife gave me an encouraging kiss on the lips as the surgery team came for me at 9 a.m. and wheeled me into the operating room. I knew that when I came out, my life would never be the same.

I survived the seven-hour surgery, where they cut out my lower esophagus and an upper portion of my stomach and then reattached what remained of these vital organs. The doctors made an incision in my belly to remove lymph nodes and insert a feeding tube. They also made an incision on the right side of my chest, between the ribs, to remove my lower esophagus and more lymph nodes. Then they brought my stomach into my chest and connected it to the remaining esophagus.

They removed a total of 24 lymph nodes.

I lay in a bed in the hospital's surgical care unit for two days following surgery. Nurses around the clock monitored my vital signs. My surgeon did not exaggerate when he said this would be the worst surgery of my life. I looked like I was at death's door. I had eight different tubes and monitors attached to my body, including an oxygen tube, a tube that went through my nose and into my esophagus, two chest tubes connected to a suction box, a catheter to empty my bladder, a feeding tube that emptied into my intestines, an epidural in my back to manage pain, and heart and blood-pressure monitors. The doctors were also afraid my lungs might collapse so every day I used an incentive spirometer, which is a small plastic device to inhale and expand my lungs. It forced me to take deep breaths.

I spent a total of fourteen days in the hospital recovering from surgery. My family was there to provide love and support for the first several days, and then it was just my wife and me to continue our journey. The doctors watched for anastomotic leaks—tissues must heal to permanently seal off where the esophagus and stomach were reattached. They told me if liquid or saliva leaked into my chest cavity, it could be fatal. I couldn't eat or drink until my tissues healed. A barium swallow test indicates the tissue had healed the anastomosis. I was ready to go home.

After they removed all the tubes and monitors from my body— except the feeding tube that I was expected to have for another month—we were on our way home to continue the recovery process. Recovering at home revealed a harsh reality. There were no doctors and nurses to care for my every need. My wife had become my sole caregiver. I took Vicodin and Percocet to manage pain, Xanax to level my anxiety, and Ambien to fall asleep at night. I was on a feeding tube 24/7 while I introduced small amounts of food into my system.

I was also on a medicine called Reglan (metoclopramide), a stomach motility stimulator. It treats gastroesophageal reflux and gastroparesis, which is a condition that affects the stomach muscles and prevents proper stomach emptying.

My stomach is now a long tube running up my chest; it is half the size of my original stomach. They cut the "flap" that keeps the insides of my stomach (mostly bile) from falling out when I bend over. I am no longer able to bend over and pick things up because the insides (bile) of my stomach will come pouring out. I sleep on an incline (about 45 degrees) to keep the bile in.

Complications

It became clear early on that I could not tolerate the feeding tube. The goal was to achieve a pump rate of 80 to 90 to get a sufficient amount of liquid food into my intestines. My highest pump rate was 50; anything exceeding 50 would result in reflux and bloating in my digestive system. Eventually, I could not even tolerate a rate of 40, so I stopped using the feeding tube. Fortunately, I was consuming enough food (calories) by mouth to justify removing the feeding tube, which doctors at Moffitt did two days later.

As fate would have it, a week later I experienced serious tremors in my legs. There were times when I could not stop my legs from shaking. I also experienced heightened anxiety and depression. These emotions spiraled out of control. Within a week, I was suicidal. My body couldn't stop shaking and I was in a constant state of anxiety. I could no longer think rationally. I would pace around the house trying to shake off the tremors while screaming to my wife that I wanted to end it.

My wife told my children about my horrific state of mind and together they convinced me to enter a mental facility at our local hospital. I felt like a fish out of water at the mental facility—it was filled with drug abusers and alcoholics. I checked out the next day but committed to seeing a psychiatrist on a weekly basis. I was put on antidepressants to help me battle my emotional demons.

Several days later, I was at the Moffitt Cancer Center for my eighth endoscopy within a fifteen-month period. The opening where they attached my esophagus to my stomach kept narrowing after the surgery, making it difficult to swallow, so during the endoscopy doctors had to continually conduct a procedure called dilation to widen the opening. This dilation problem was a complication from my original surgery. We met with the gastroenterologist before the procedure and told him about my severe tremors and anxiety. Without hesitation, he told me to stop taking the drug Reglan. He said tremors and anxiety and deep depression are the primary side effects of Reglan.

As if he had waved a magic wand—within days the tremors, anxiety, depression, and suicidal thoughts vanished. It was the Reglan. I had heard how side effects of many medications negatively affect the lives of millions of senior citizens, and now I had experienced it firsthand. Going forward, I would always read about the possible side effects of every medication prescribed for me.

Upon reflection, no coping skills helped me deal with the emotional basket of tremors, anxiety, depression, and suicidal thoughts. I was too far gone and too irrational to apply coping methods. At some point, constant suffering overcomes the ability to cope. I hope this never happens to me again.

Getting off Reglan created a new set of problems for me. Without Reglan, the motility of my stomach (the ability to digest and move the food) weakened considerably. I was no longer able to consume food by mouth. Within two weeks, I lost seven pounds and checked back into the Moffitt Cancer Center Hospital.

I stayed at the hospital for twelve days. It was obvious I had serious complications from the surgery. Most patients recovering from an esophagectomy eventually regain the ability to eat five or six small meals per day. They regain muscle movement (motility) throughout their digestive system. The organs of the digestive system contain muscles that enable the digestive walls to move. The movement of organ walls propels food and liquid. Movement of the esophagus, stomach, and intestine is called peristalsis. My digestive system was seriously compromised.

My stomach's ability to move food to my intestines stopped working. Doctors inserted another feeding tube to bring food directly to my intestines from a pump outside my body. But I couldn't tolerate the feeding tube and again experienced reflux, bile, and bloating problems every day, which diminished my quality of life. Some days I woke up gagging and vomiting. The doctors didn't know why my stomach stopped working and hoped one day it would function again. My intestines were also not working efficiently, which was probably why I couldn't tolerate the feeding tube that poured liquid food into my intestines.

I tried to maintain a positive attitude, but I wasn't able to tolerate the feeding tube. The feeding tube created most of my health issues. Living in the present moment meant living with the not-so-gentle suffering of weight loss, reflux, bloating, bile, coughing, gagging, vomiting, depression, and fatigue.

I returned to the hospital for ten more days. There was a frustration that my doctors and my wife and I didn't know what to do about. At first, the doctors thought I couldn't handle my reduced quality of life. One doctor even suggested that I see a psychiatrist to cope with my health issues. After a number of examinations, the doctors concluded that my stomach and intestines were not working, which is why I couldn't tolerate my feeding tube.

The doctors decided to take me off the feeding tube and all other food and liquids. The objective was to completely empty my stomach and intestines, which would take four days of no food or liquids. I was intravenously fed sugar water, but that was it. I lost six pounds during my hospital stay. They basically wanted to empty my stomach and intestines and start over.

I was sent home with a new feeding tube formula that the doctors hoped my digestive system would tolerate. The very first day on the feeding tube, I gagged and then vomited. I had reached my limit and took myself off the feeding tube. I would never be on a feeding tube again—I don't care if I become emaciated. Never again would I endure the constant reflux, bile, bloating, gagging, coughing, and vomiting.

Without the feeding tube, I drank Boost Plus, which has 360 calories per 8 ounces. Some days I consumed 1,400 calories per day and some days I was able to consume 2,000.

It was a liquid diet—would it be forever? Would I ever be able to eat real food again?

I was desperate to find a medicine that works like Reglan without the side effects. One of the doctors at Moffitt recommends the drug domperidone. It is not legal in the United States, so I use a Canadian pharmacy to acquire the medicine. After several weeks, it didn't seem to work well, but I continued to take it, nevertheless. At least there were no side effects.

The reality of the situation stared me in the face. This was my life now—I lived on a liquid diet. I was fifteen pounds under my normal weight. I needed to accept this new reality and get on with my life. I needed to accept that the complications from surgery wouldn't go away. I had to overcome my physical limitations by focusing and strengthening my spirit.

I went through a time of pretending: pretending that was normal, pretending that the cancer and my complications would go away. Finally, I realized that I had to reverse pivot, avoid negativity, and become more positive.

I had been through real suffering: uncontrollable physical tremors, vomiting, depression, and suicidal thoughts. Real suffering is different from enduring the marks of aging. I understand someone wanting to end his or her life to avoid painful constant suffering. Thankfully, I was past that stage. I must now accept, adapt, and appreciate a new way of life, even if it's a lower quality of life. I must possess the right attitude toward my new life. I must learn to live with a liquid diet and reflux and occasional gagging and vomiting. I can do this.

To add fuel to the fire, a recent CT scan (computerized tomography) had detected nodules in my thyroid. The thyroid makes hormones that regulate how your body uses energy and help your body function normally. After a biopsy, I was diagnosed with papillary thyroid cancer. I would have surgery to remove my thyroid. Compared to esophageal cancer, thyroid cancer is minor league, so, in the spirit of positivity, I treated it as an inconvenience.

Mayo Clinic

The doctors at the Moffitt Cancer Center had done all they could for me. They specialize in cancer, not stomach/intestinal motility complications. I would continue to visit Moffitt for semiannual exams and scans that would look for signs of cancer rearing its ugly head again.

My next stop was the Mayo Clinic in Jacksonville, Florida, where doctors specialize in digestive motility problems. Was there another new drug for me that would improve my digestive motility? How many more endoscopies would I undergo? I had already undergone eight endoscopies with the accompanying anesthesia. Anesthesia is a state of controlled, temporary loss of sensation or awareness that is induced for medical purposes (i.e., surgery). It often induces or maintains unconsciousness, which could result in memory loss or cognitive dysfunction. I anxiously underwent an unheard-of ninth endoscopy and anesthesia within an eighteen-month period, and the doctor found nothing to explain my motility problems.

But the doctor recommended that I try the drug Reglan again. Remember that Reglan's side effects were horrendous for me. It sent me into a deep depression and gave me serious body tremors. His reasoning was that Reglan was the only drug that improved my stomach's motility and permitted me to eat solid food, so we need to work with Reglan and minimize its negative side effects. His approach was to keep me on Reglan for only two weeks, then take me off it for two weeks, then back on Reglan for two weeks and then off it for two weeks—so on and so on.

The stars were finally aligned for me—the two weeks off and two weeks on Reglan worked! I was able to eat solid food while on Reglan.

And when I was off it, I was still able to eat solid food. It seems like the Reglan continued to work through my system during the weeks that I was not on it.

I followed the on again/off again Reglan plan religiously for about six months, and then, miraculously, I no longer needed the Reglan. It seemed that the on again/off again method eventually triggered my motility system to work again, freeing me of the need to take Reglan.

I've gained most of my weight back and I follow a restricted food diet (which excludes hard-to-digest foods like steak and pork). I continue to sleep on a 45-degree angle. Post-surgery has also left me with a permanent "tickle" in my esophagus that, at times, results in persistent coughing (and sometimes gagging) for prolonged periods.

Final Thoughts

When I'm contemplative, I think about my temporary existence on this planet. We are all dying; some of us will go sooner than others. I think about how civilization advances and how I will soon miss the future. We all miss the party, so to speak. We only experience progress as a collective evolutionary group of humans. We are all left out of long-term progress.

Time is passing me by, and it may soon be time to pass the baton to younger generations. Humans' willingness to pass the baton is our survival instinct at work. Without willingness, we would go down fighting like a crazed tiger with its back to the wall. This is not a civil thing to do in the face of inevitability.

Am I envious of my peers who may outlive me by 20 to 30 years? No, because we all confront finality, and in the big scheme of things life is just the blink of an eye. We are just a spec of matter; we are here in earthly existence for just a split second in universal time until we dissipate and dissolve as splattered energy into the universe. Sometimes heavy thoughts consume me.

I think about all the people who lived and died before me. On a personal level I think about Grandpa and Nona and Uncle Fred, and my dad, who passed away as of this writing: Where did they go? Are they just nothingness, or are they somewhere in an afterlife? I think about celebrities who fall off the cliff one by one. I think about old movies like *It's a Wonderful Life*: James Stewart, Donna Reed, and all the cast members are gone. I think about the great professional athletes of my childhood: Mickey Mantle, Roger Maris, Muhammad Ali—gone. The inevitability of change is the changing of the guard for humans.

Perhaps the biggest challenge facing me is loss of control. When you know that aging and death are inevitable, you feel you are losing a grip on life. That is a tough one to handle. The bottom line is that my cancer has given me a new appreciation for growing old.

Acknowledgments

Writing a book about a personal journey of crisis is a surreal as well as therapeutic process. Fortunately, my battle against cancer led me to embrace a positive mindset about life and aging. I hope telling my story helps others discover the extraordinary power of positive aging.

I earned a doctorate in economics, not gerontology, so I am not an expert on the intricacies of aging. I owe a debt of gratitude to all those professionals and organizations who have been dedicated to advancing our knowledge about how to grow old successfully.

This book would not be possible without the help of others. I'm eternally grateful to my medical team at the Moffitt Cancer Center, especially Dr. Jacques-Pierre Fontaine, Joe Garret, ARNP, and Dr. Sarah Hoffe. I am cancer-free today because of them.

I am deeply grateful for the love and support of my wife, Carole, who held me close throughout my arduous journey. And to my children—Abbey, Jeff and Jenna—and to my parents, and siblings for their caring and loving ways.

I am forever indebted to my publisher, Kent Sorsky, and editor, Tammy Ditmore for their editorial help and keen insight in bringing my journey to life. Very special thanks also go to those who offered helpful comments on various drafts of this book: Bob Sperling, Susan Landeis, Angela Gentile, Linda Mosley, and Mary Furlong. A shout-out to Jaguar Bennett for his strong guidance on the promotion of my book.

Finally, to all those wonderful and inspiring senior citizens on my Meals on Wheels route and my Friends for Seniors program at United We Age—thank you so much for allowing me into your lives. You have given me greater clarity about how to age with grace, dignity, and joy.

Notes

1. Sources: AARP and the U.S. Census Bureau Forecasts, Haver Analytics, all from Duetsche Bank Research, Global Research, November 2018.

2. Valerie Gladwell, School of Biological Sciences, Researchgate.net, University of Essex, "Beat your Body Clock," Men's Health, August 8, 2013, menshealth.com.

3. Courtney Reyers, "The Depression Boom: As U.S. Population Ages, Mental Illness Rises," March 13, 2013, National Alliance on Mental Illness: www.nami.org/About-NAMI/NAMI-News/2013/The-Depression-Boom-As-US-Population-Ages-Mental.

4. Elizabeth Phelan and Eric Larson, "Successful Aging—Where Next?"; Journal of the American Geriatrics Society, August 2002, Volume 50, Issue 7.

5. Elizabeth Phelan, Lynda Anderson, Andrea Lacroix, Eric Larson, "Older Adults' View of Successful Aging," Journal of the American Geriatrics Society, January 22, 2004, Vol 52, Issue 2.

6. Kori Miller, "What Is Positive Aging? 10 Tips to Promote the Positive Aspects of Aging," Positive Psychology.com, May 2019. positivepsychology.com/positive-aging/

7. Lewina Lee, Peter James, Emily Zevon, Eric Kim, Claudia Trudel-Fitzgerald, Aoron Spiroill, Francine Grodstein and Laura Kubzansky, "Optimism Is Associated with Exceptional Longevity in 2 Epidemiologic Cohorts of Men & Women," September 10, 2019, PNAS: Proceedings of the National Academy of Sciences.

8. CW Greider, "Telomeres and Senesence: The History, the Experiment, the Future," Current Biology, 1998, 8:R 178-81 (PubMed) (Google Scholar).

JW Szostak and EH Blackburn, "Cloning Yeast Telomeres on Linear Plasmid Vectors," Cell, 1982, 29, 245-255.

CW Greider, EH Blackburn, "A Telomeric Sequence in the RNA of Tetrahymena Telomerase Required for Telomere Repeat Synthesis," Nature, 1989, 337; 331-7.

CW Greider and EH Blackburn, "Identification of a Specific Telomere Terminal Transferase Activity inTetrahymena Extracts," Cell, 1985; 43; 405-13.

9. "What Is a Telomere? Human Cellular Aging", TA-65, TA Sciences, tasciences.com/what-is-a-telomere.html.

10. Richard Cawthon, "Are Telomeres the Key to Aging and Cancer?" 2002, Learn.Genetics.utah.edu.

11. Ellissa Epel and Elizabeth Blackburn, The Telomere Effect: A Revolutionary Approach to Living Younger, Healthier, Longer, Grand Central Publishing, January 3, 2017.

Ellissa Epel and Arie Prather, "Stress, Telomeres and Psychopathology: Toward Deeper Understanding of a Triad of Early Aging," The Annual Review of Clinical Psychology, 2018, clinpsy.annualrreviews.org.

Ellissa Epel, "How to Create the Ideal Diet for Telomere Health," February 13, 2017, Elle.com.

12. Becca Levy, The Longitudinal Study in the Journal of Personality and Social Psychology (vol 83, No. 2, 2002).

13. 2014 General Social Survey, National Opinion Research Center, Funded by National Science Foundation, 2014, thearda.com.

14. "What Is Positive Mindset: 89 Ways to Achieve Positive Mental Attitude," Courtney Ackerman, May 7, 2018, Positivepsychology.com.

15. Everything Psychology Book, Kendra Cherry, Adams Publishing, 2010.

16. "There Are 50,000 Thoughts Standing Between You and Your Partner Every Day," Bruce Davis, PhD, Huffington Post Blog, July 23, 2013.

17. The Grant Study of Adult Development, begun in 1938, George E. Valliant, Principal Investigator, Harvard University Press, October 30, 2012, Harvard Medical School.

18. Macmillan Cancer Support Study: Facing the Fight Alone: Cancer, Isolation and Loneliness, July 2014, Ciaran Devane, Chief Executive, macmillan.org.uk. Lonely Cancer Patients Failing to Complete Treatment, Charity Claims, Charlie Cooper, August 2014, Independent.co.uk.

19. The Kaiser Foundation Study, United States, United Kingdom & Japan: An International Study, by Bianca Di Julio, Liz Hamel, Cailey Muhana, and Mollyann Brodie, August 30, 2018, KFF.org. Different Approaches to Recognizing Loneliness in the Elderly, Judith Graham, Kaiser Health News, March 17, 2019, ABCnews.go.com.

20. Linda Fried testimony to an ad hoc committee under the auspices of the National Academies of Sciences, 2018, nationalacademies.org/projectandactivities

21. "Expectations Regarding Aging, Physical Activity, and Physical Function in Older Adults," Aili Breda and Amber Watts, Gerontology and Geriatric Medicine, February 27, 2017, NCBI.NLM.NIH.gov.

22. The Paradox of Choice, Barry Schwartz, Harper Perennial Publishers, 2004 (Barry Schwartz, TED Talk July 2005, England, YouTube.com).

23. Dean Rosson, CEO Executive Seminar, Vistage Meeting, November 12, 2019, deanrosson.com.

24. National Cancer Institute of the National Institutes of Health, Cancer. gov/commoncancertypes, American Cancer Society, Cancer Facts and Figures, February 21, 2019.

25. G Livingston, A Smoerlad, V Orgeta, S Costafreda, J Huntley, D Ames, "Dementia Prevention, Intervention, and Care," The Lancet Commissions, Vol 390, Issue 10113, pp. 2673-2734, December 16, 2017.

26. "Retirement Causes a Major Decline in Physical and Mental Health," New Research Finds, May 16, 2013, Institute of Economic Affairs, Media Post, iea.org.uk.

27. "Muffled Hearing: Health Issues That Can Cause Hearing Loss," WebMD, August 1, 2018, WebMD.com/healthyAging.Reference.

28. "7 Celebrities Embracing Wrinkles and Destabilizing Growing Older," October 13, 2015, Bustle.com.

29. Julia Roberts Quotes, BrainyQuotes.com.

30. Owen Jarus, "20 of the Worst Epidemics and Pandemics in History," Live Science, March 21, 2020, www.livescience.com/worst-epidemics-and-pandemics-in-history.html

31. Susan Sarandon, Brainy Quote, www.brainyquote.com/quotes/susan_sarandon_126075.

32. Elizabeth Kubler-Ross, On Death and Dying, Simon and Schuster, 1969.

33. Steve Jobs Quote, Goodreads.com.

34. Woody Allen, Wood Allen Quotes, BrainyQuotes.com.

35. Could It Be B12?: An Epidemic of Misdiagnoses, 2nd Edition, Sally M. Pacholok, RN, and Jeffrey J. Stuart, DO, Quill Driver Books, 2011.

36. en.wikipedia.org/wiki/Emotional_intelligence

37. "Measure EI for Employee Development with the EQ-I 2.0 Assessment," Upward Solutions, Upwardsolutionscc.com.

38. "Stress Management—A Master Class: An Inaugural Lecture," Stephen Palmer, Counselling Psychology Review, 16, 1, 18-27, November 1, 2000, academia.edu.

39. Daniel Goleman, Emotional Intelligence: Why It Can Matter More than IQ, Bantam Books, 1995.

40. Adopt a Senior, Jackson, New Jersey, adopt-a-senior.org/home

41. 2018 Profile of Older Americans, Administration for Community Living (and Administration on Aging), Division of Department of Health and Human Services, April 2019, acl.gov/aging-and-disability-in-america/data-and-research/profile-older-americans

42. Macmillan Cancer Support Study: "Facing the Fight Alone: Cancer, Isolation and Loneliness," July 2014, Ciaran Devane, Chief Executive, macmillan.org.uk. "Lonely Cancer Patients Failing to Complete Treatment, Charity Claims," Charlie Cooper, August 2014, Independent.co.uk

43. "Marriage Linked to Lower Heart Risks," NYU Lagone Medical Center study (2014) presented to the American College of Cardiology, March 29, 2014.

44. Home Care Financial Assistance and Payment Options, July 2019, PayforSeniorcare.com.

45. Jack O'Brien, "Immigrants Comprise More Than 18% of Healthcare Workers," June 3, 2019, The Institute of Medicine, National Academies of Sciences, ihi.org.

46. "Families Caring for an Aging America," The National Academies of Sciences, September 13, 2016, National Academies Press, nap.edu.

47. Caregiving in the U.S. 2015 Report, Public Policy Institute, AARP, aarp.org.

48. "Social Isolation, Loneliness and All-Cause Mortality in Older Men and Women," by Andrew Steptoe, Aparna Shankar, Panaytes Demakakos, and Jane Wardle, Department of Epidemiology and Public Health, University College London, February 15, 2013.

49. "A Social Psychological Perspective on the Stigmatization of Older Adults," by Becca Levy, Journal of Personality and Social Psychology (vol 83, No.2, 2002).

50. "Contact Hypothesis and Inter-Age Attitudes: A Field Study of Cross-Age Contact," Ayshalom Caspi, Social Psychology Quarterly, Vol 47, No 1 (March 1984).

51. "On the Malleability of Automatic Attitudes: Combating Automatic Prejudice with Images of Admired and Disliked Individuals," Nilanjana Dasgupta and Anthony Greenwald, Journal of Personality and Social Psychology 81 (5), 2001.

52. "Life Stress, Social Support and Self-Esteem in an Elderly Population," N. Krause, 1987, APA PsycNET, psycnet.apa.org.

Index

Index

meditation, 7, 25, 29, 39, 43–45, 54, 145, 165–166, 172, 177, 182, 185, 186
  apps, 45, 187
  deep, 44–45
  duration, 40, 44
  failed, 44
  groups, 22
  process, 40, 44
  simple, 44, 166, 170, 173, 178
memory loss, 18, 89, 140, 177, 178, 186, 187–188
mental health, 15, 47, 73, 86, 89, 164
  lifestyle plan for, 177–180
Middle East respiratory syndrome (MERS), 118
Miller, Keri, 4
mind, 24–25
  state of, 25
  stimulating, 34–36, 149, 165
  upper, 25
mindfulness, 14–16, 29, 39–47, 49, 57, 71, 158, 181, 182
  definition of, 39, 40
  exception to, 47
  teachings, 41–42
Mintzer, Dorian, 4
Mirren, Helen, 116
"Miss Mary," 64
mobility, declining, 2, 12, 14, 18, 85, 88, 105–109, 130, 174
  consequences of, 106
  coping with, 108–109
  devices, 107–108
  treatment for, 106
mobility scooter, 60, 105, 107–108
Monroe, Robert, 30
Mortality, facing, 10
multiple sclerosis, 14, 181
multitasking, 45, 167, 178

music, 35, 170, 172, 179, 183
  loud, 110–111
Mutzner, Ruth, 4

N

National Academy of Sciences, 67, 193
National Association of Realtors, 42
National Institute on Aging, 4, 66
National Senior Citizens Day, 203
negativity, 16, 37, 50, 53, 54, 77
New Age beliefs, 14, 25, 133, 135, 183
New York Fire Patrol, 63
New York Times, 103
New York University Lagone Medical Center, 193
Newhouse, Meg, 4
Nobel Prize, 6
note/memory calendar, 179, 180

O

Oculus Go Standalone VR Hea, 187
Oculus Quest All-in-One VR Gaming Headset, 187
"Old Age Appreciated: The Positive Aging Movement," 4
optimism, 6, 33, 146
organized, being, 79, 167
osteoporosis, 87, 141
out-of-body experiences (OBE), 29–32, 182, 185–186, 187

P

Page, Jimmy, 110
Palmer, Stephen, 145
Paradox of Choice, The (Schwartz), 74

Parkinson's Disease, 14, 73–74, 85, 87, 157, 168, 181, 184
peaceful moments, seeking, 28–29, 165, 173, 182
perspective, 59–60, 148
Phelan, Elizabeth, 2
physical therapy, 106
pneumonia, 87
positive aging, 2–3
  benefits of, 4–5, 11
  lifestyle plan for, 162–190
  lifestyle, why it works, 162–163l
  movement, 4
  road map to, 13–17
  science of, 5–7
Positive Aging Room, 10–12, 16, 129, 151, 162–163
PositivePsychology.com, 4, 49
positivity, 15, 16, 17, 49–56, 57, 71, 158, 167
  definition, 49
  embracing, 12
  exhibiting, 77
  focus on, 53–54
  mindset, 3
  practicing, 3, 50–55
possibilities, 75, 97, 168
post-surgery life, 1, 78, 151, 152
Power of Now, 133, 135
Power of Now, The (Tolle), 41–42
Power of Positive Aging program, 23
Practical Aging Room, 10, 11, 12–13, 129, 162, 163
Prather, Arie, 7
prayer, 33–34, 124, 165, 182
present, living in the, 3, 16, 20, 39, 43–47, 49, 75, 95, 97, 112, 123–125, 167, 171–172, 174–175

About the Author

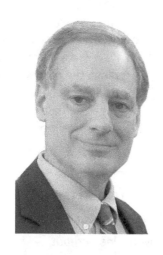

David Lereah is an economist, cancer survivor, motivational speaker, and founder of the nonprofit organization United We Age. He previously was the chief economist for the National Association of Realtors and the Mortgage Bankers Association. He is the author of four books, the most recent being *All Real Estate Is Local*. Lereah's economic commentary has regularly appeared in the *Wall Street Journal*, the *New York Times*, and *Business Week*, and on CNN, CNBC, and other media. Lereah began his career on the faculties of the Univeristy of Virginia and Rutgers Univeristy. He earned his PhD in Economics from the University of Virginia. Lereah lives in Port St. Lucie, Florida.

Better Living in Later Life
with Dr. Ruth Westheimer

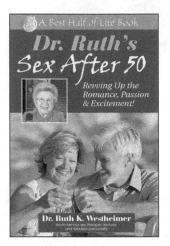

$14.95
Paperback

Dr. Ruth's Sex After 50

Revving Up the Romance, Passion and Excitement!
by Dr. Ruth Westheimer

Many people enjoy the best sex of their lives after 50! Sure, with aging comes physical and psychological changes, but the misconceptions and inappropriate attitudes developed over the years about the natural aging process may cause more damage to a couple's sex life than anything physical. Dr. Ruth K. Westheimer, world-famous sex therapist, guides the reader through the physical and emotional challenges of sex after 50, revving up the romance, passion and excitement as only Dr. Ruth knows how!

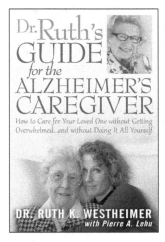

$16.95
Paperback

Dr. Ruth's Guide for the Alzheimer's Caregiver

How to Care for Your Loved One without Getting Overwhelmed ... and without Doing It All Yourself
by Dr. Ruth K. Westheimer
with Pierre A. Lehu

America's most-trusted sex therapist brings much-needed help to overburdened caregivers! **Dr. Ruth's Guide for the Alzheimer's Caregiver** presents coping strategies for both the practical problems and emotional stresses of Alzheimer's care. Dr. Ruth shows you how to avoid caregiver burnout; get effective support from family and friends; deal effectively with doctors, care providers and facilities.

Stay Active, Stay Healthy
with Dr. Joan Vernikos

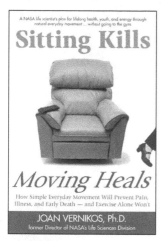

$14.95
Paperback

Sitting Kills, Moving Heals
How Simple Everyday Movement Will Prevent Pain, Illness, and Early Death—and Exercise Alone Won't
by Joan Vernikos, Ph.D., former Director of NASA's Life Sciences Division

New medical research has shown that sitting too much will shorten your life, even if you get regular exercise. *Sitting Kills, Moving Heals* shows that the key to lifelong fitness and good health is constant, nonstrenuous movement that resists the force of gravity. This easy-to-follow, common-sense plan will show you how simple, everyday, and fun activities like walking, gardening, dancing, golf, and more will keep you fit, strong and independent your whole life long.

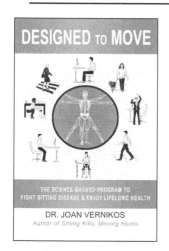

$12.95
Paperback

Designed to Move
The Science-Backed Program to Fight Sitting Disease and Enjoy Lifelong Health
by Dr. Joan Vernikos

Science has proven that prolonged sitting is terrible for your health. In *Designed to Move*, Dr. Joan Vernikos, former director of NASA's Life Sciences Division, presents a scientific exercise plan to reverse the effects of prolonged sitting through simple, low-impact, frequent movement, ideal for office workers and others who sit too much. Vernikos explains why frequent movement that resists the force of gravity is essential for good health offers easy exercises to add gravity-resistant movement throughout the day that can be done in any office, workplace, or home.

Available from bookstores, online bookstores, and QuillDriverBooks.com, or by calling toll-free 1-800-345-4447.